Further Statistics in Dentistry

Further Statistics in Dentistry

Aviva Petrie
Senior Lecturer in Statistics,
Eastman Dental Institute for Oral Health Care Sciences,
University College London
Honorary Lecturer,
Department of Medical Statistics,
London School of Hygiene and Tropical Medicine

John Bulman
Honorary Reader in Dental Public Health,
Eastman Dental Institute for Oral Health Care Sciences,
University College London

John Osborn
Professor of Epidemiological Methods,
Department of Public Health Sciences
Università di Roma 'La Sapienza'

2002

Published by the British Dental Association
64 Wimpole Street, London, W1G 8YS

Preface

It is now some thirteen years since our first offering, *Statistics in Dentistry,* appeared in print. Both the authors of that earlier work had been involved for many years in introducing statistics to dentists, and had recognised the existence of an increasing awareness among dentists of the need for and the advantages of a working knowledge of statistical techniques. Furthermore, existing textbooks, while in other respects admirable, lacked examples in the dental field and usually did not address the specific statistical problems likely to confront dentists. Nevertheless, we had our doubts concerning the viability of producing yet another statistical textbook, and it was really due to the enthusiastic support and encouragement of Dame Margaret Seward, who was then Editor of the *British Dental Journal,* that the project was finally launched. Dame Margaret's judgement has since been vindicated, as demonstrated by the sales of the book to date, and, with increasing numbers of General Dental Practitioners becoming involved in research projects within their practices, the demand for it looks set to continue.

One of the premises upon which that first book was based was that dentists, like doctors, could not normally be expected to have any marked mathematical aptitude (if they had, they would probably be mathematicians rather than dentists). For this reason we deliberately tried to simplify our approach and avoid any taint of statistical jargon whenever we could. In other words, we stuck firmly to basics and tried to be practical rather than theoretical. However, in recent years and on many occasions at dental meetings, I have been approached by dentists saying, in effect, 'Your book is fine as far as it goes, but I'd like to learn more, so where should I go now?' This new book is really our attempt to provide an answer to this question for such colleagues.

Once again we are grateful to the Editor of the *British Dental Journal*, Mike Grace, Margaret Seward's successor, for smoothing our path, together with an old friend, Stephen Hancocks, O.B.E., the *Journal*'s Commissioning Editor. Discerning readers will note that we have added a new author for this second book. Of the original authors, the one writing this Preface is fast approaching his three-score years and ten, while the other is heavily committed, as a Professor of Epidemiological Methods, to teaching and research at one of the largest medical schools in Italy. We therefore felt that new blood could only be advantageous. We had both known, worked with, and respected the expertise of Aviva Petrie over many years. She, too, has been involved in teaching statistics to dentists, as well as to those in the medical and veterinary professions, and she has also written her own textbooks, so she was well aware of what she was taking on. We were therefore delighted when she agreed to join the team, and we both agree that she has taken on the lion's share to bring this work to fruition.

At this point, we should perhaps stress that this new book is not intended in any way to replace the old one. We would submit that *Statistics in Dentistry* still provides the basic techniques which should satisfy the needs of the majority of dentists embarking on their own research projects or, alternatively, wishing to check the statistical analysis (or lack of it) in papers published in the professional journals. But for those who have been bitten by the statistical bug and wish to know more, or those who have to cope with special statistical problems, we hope our new offering will be useful. By its very nature, we do not really expect that it will appeal to as wide a readership as *Statistics in Dentistry*, but we do hope that it will fill a gap which has existed in the available dental statistical literature.

John Bulman

Acknowledgements

As well as those individuals mentioned in the Preface, the authors would like to acknowledge the help and co-operation received from Peter Fyne, Assistant Editor of the *British Dental Journal*, and thank him for his infinite patience at the proof-reading stage of the book. It is rarely possible to totally separate family and work, and so we take this opportunity to include in this acknowledgement the parts played by our spouses, Gerald, Judith and Angela, and our children, Nina, Andrew and Karen, and Vivian and Tom. Finally, we are grateful to the students we have taught over the years who have kept us focused and from whom we continue to learn.

ISBN 0 904588 74 2

Printed and bound by
Dennis Barber Limited,
Lowestoft, Suffolk

Contents

Research designs 1

This book is designed to supplement, rather than replace, the material contained in the earlier series on statistics in dentistry published in the *British Dental Journal* and subsequently made available in book form.[1] With the increasing availability of calculators, personal computers and computer statistical software packages, the need for details of the 'nuts and bolts' of statistical theory has diminished, but the need for an understanding of how and when such theory should be applied, and how studies should be designed to make best use of it, has probably increased. It is with these thoughts in mind that this new book is being offered.

Definitions

Inevitably every specialist subject has its own vocabulary, where often everyday words take on a special meaning. These new meanings are usually designed to put across a specific and frequently used concept, and therefore it is useful for the novice to be aware of and understand them. Unfortunately, statisticians, like specialists in other disciplines, have not avoided the use of jargon, or words apparently invented to make a simple idea incomprehensible to the outsider. Here, then, are some of the terms and ideas which are employed regularly in any statistical investigation.

Variables, Factors and Effects

A **variable** is a quantity that can take different values for individuals in a study; it is called a **response variable** when it relates to the outcome of interest. A variable may be *quantitative*, that is, it takes a *numerical value*; or it may be *qualitative* or *categorical*, in which case it describes an attribute. For example, changes in body weight after specific periods on a prescribed diet are quantitative because, for each subject, the observation takes a numerical value. In contrast, a child may or may not show evidence of dental caries at a particular moment in time. In this case the observation describes the presence or absence of a characteristic, and it is therefore qualitative rather than quantitative. When the values for the variable for several individual subjects are aggregated, quantitative observations may be summarised to yield some sort of average value, for example the arithmetic mean. Qualitative data, particularly if related to disease or death, may be summarised by a proportion or a rate, such as the prevalence or incidence rate. All these summary measures which represent characteristics of the observations in the population are called **parameters.**

Although it is possible to define the term **factor** in a number of ways, it most commonly refers to a quantity which is a possible cause of variation of the outcome of interest in an investigation. If the factor is a categorical variable, then the different categories are called **levels** of the factor. For example, in a clinical trial, the factor 'treatment' with two levels would divide the group under investigation into two subgroups, such as those who receive an active treatment and those who do not. (Note however, in statistics, the word 'treatment' does not necessarily mean a treatment as given by a doctor or dentist to a patient. It is used in a more general sense to mean any experimental procedure applied to any experimental unit). The factor 'gender' divides the subjects into males and females; the factor 'age' can be used to divide the study group into different age categories.

The **effect** of a factor can be determined by estimating the appropriate parameter, such as the average or proportion, for each level of the factor and then comparing the resulting estimates. This is just a clumsy way of saying, for example, that social class (the factor) has an effect on caries incidence rate (the parameter) if the latter increases with decreasing social class (each social class specifies a level of the factor). As another example, the effect of the factor 'topical fluoride' may be different in the average annual caries increment in those subjects who receive it (one level of the factor) and in those who do not (a second level of the factor). For a particular study, the effect of the factor 'gender' may be that males have twice the risk of getting the disease than females. If the factor of interest is a health intervention (eg a new treatment), then the effect of the health intervention is of primary interest; ie it is necessary to compare the response variable in those 'exposed' to the intervention with those who are not. Those subjects who do not receive the intervention are often called a 'control' or 'comparison' group, which may nevertheless comprise those who are on a standard treatment (or a placebo). Such comparisons are sometimes made by examining for each individual the response variable, say the area of an oral lesion, before and after the exposure to the intervention and then comparing these differences between groups. A study that has no control group is, in general, an unsatisfactory way of investigating the effect of a factor and is often called an **uncontrolled case series**.

Interaction

Very often in a study there will be factors, other than just the principal factor of interest, which have an effect on the response. Suppose a study is designed to investigate the effect of a particular health intervention. The study population is divided into two groups, those who are exposed to the intervention and those who are not; ie the factor 'intervention' has two levels. Suppose also that the study includes both males and females so that the factor 'gender' also has two levels. An **interaction** between the factors exists if the effect of the intervention in males differs from the effect of the intervention in females. Interaction is sometimes called 'effect modification' because the effect of one factor is modified or changed by the level of the other. If an important interaction exists, it does not make much sense to speak of the effect of the factor of interest without specifying the level of the other. An extreme example would be an intervention which is beneficial to one half of the population but harmful to the other half. It would not be very useful to report that on average the intervention had no effect. A more realistic example might be a study specifically designed to determine those sectors of a population who might gain greatest benefit, thus enabling appropriate targeting of the intervention.

Confounding

In 1948, the year the National Health Service was introduced in the United Kingdom, the crude death rate was 11·0 per 1,000 population in England and Wales. This implies that on average about eleven people died per annum for every thousand people in the population. Since then, the rate has increased slowly and erratically, and for example in 1986 it was 11·6 per 1,000. In other words, the rate of dying seems to have increased since the introduction of the NHS. But the observed effect of the introduction of the National Health Service is distorted if there exists some other factor, for example age, which is associated with the death rate, and which is distributed unequally in the years being compared. Since the proportion of the population who are elderly increased during the 38 years between 1948 and 1986, it is not surprising that the crude death rate did not continue to decline from its minimum ever value of 11·0 in 1948. So although the apparent effect of the introduction of the National Health Service has been an increase in the crude death rate, this apparent effect has been distorted by the factor 'age', and the effect of the intervention is said to be **confounded** or confused by 'age'. Using the same reasoning, just because over a period of time per capita sugar consumption in a country decreased with a parallel decrease in dental caries, it should not be assumed that the reduced sugar consumption caused the decrease in caries. There might, for example, have been increased availability of fluoride dentifrices over the same period, and this could be the confounding variable which was the main reason for the fall in caries.

Bias

The considerations which govern a well designed study rely, to a large extent, on ensuring that the study is free from bias. Bias is present when the results from the study are systematically distorted and so are consistently above (or below) what they should be. Biases may arise in a number of ways. Typical examples are:

- *Observer bias* — when one observer consistently over-reports (or under-reports) a variable. This may be resolved by training and calibration.

- *Selection bias* — when the individuals in the study are not representative of the population of interest. This may be avoided by ensuring that a random method of selection is used rather than relying on purposive or judgement sampling, where investigators include in their samples those individuals who they believe are typical or representative of the population.

- *Publication bias* — which is a tendency for journals to publish only 'significant' results.

- *Recall bias* — when certain patients have a differential ability to remember details about their past.

- *Allocation bias* — when treatment groups in an experimental study are not comparable with respect to the variables influencing the response of

4

interest. Random allocation (also called *randomisation*) of the treatments to the patients is a way of avoiding this bias and is discussed in detail in the first chapter on clinical trials.

- *Assessment bias* — resulting from the manner in which the responses to treatment are assessed, often because of the subjective nature of those responses and the preconceived notions of those assessing the response. Making the trial 'blind' so that the study personnel and perhaps the patients are unaware of which treatment each patient receives is a way of overcoming assessment bias. This is discussed in more detail in Chapter 3 — Clinical Trials 1.

Statistical inference

In many situations, investigators are interested in the effect of some 'intervention' or 'treatment' in a particular target population. For example, the question of interest might be, 'What effect would the introduction of water fluoridated at 1 ppm have on the prevalence of dental caries in Salisbury?' To answer this question, exactly as phrased, would involve studying the whole population of Salisbury before and after the introduction of fluoridated water. In practice, the investigators might decide to study the effect of the intervention on a small scale by looking at a representative sample of the population, rather than the whole population. If the effect of the intervention were beneficial in the small scale sample study, an **inference** might be made that the effect of the intervention would be beneficial in the whole population. Clearly such an inference might not be exactly correct; the effect in the whole population may be greater or less than the effect in the sample. Indeed, the observed effect in the sample will depend on precisely which sample is used for the study. Different samples will give slightly different estimates of the effect of the intervention in the population, although common sense will suggest that the larger the sample, the more likely will the effect approximate closely to the effect in the population. Thus any particular sample study is likely to have some degree of **sampling error** if the effect of the intervention in the sample is used to estimate the effect of the intervention in the whole population. Statistical inference is, to a large extent, concerned with **estimating the magnitude of an effect** in a population and assessing the sampling error of the estimate, using evidence obtained from a representative sample drawn from that population. The second major component of statistical inference involves *assessing the effects of interest*, achieved by performing **significance tests**, also called **hypothesis tests**.

Estimation

In estimation, the sample study provides an estimate of the effect of the intervention in the population and consideration of sampling error yields an interval, known as a **confidence interval**, which is reasonably certain to contain the (unknown) true population effect. For example, suppose a sample study implied that fluoridated drinking water in a given area would halve exactly the incidence of dental caries in 12-year-old children. If this sample result were extended to the population there would clearly be some doubt as to whether the incidence of caries would be halved exactly. However, statistical analysis of the sample data might lead the investigators to be reasonably certain that the effect of fluoridated water would be to reduce the incidence in the population to between 40% and 60% of the pre-intervention level. This interval, which is believed to include the true effect of the intervention in the population, is called a confidence interval, and the degree of belief is measured by a probability expressed as a percentage, usually 95%. Thus a 95% confidence interval for the effect of an intervention is commonly interpreted to mean that there is a 95% chance that the interval will include the true (but unknown) population effect of the intervention.

Hypothesis tests

A hypothesis test is concerned with answering a simple question about the effect of interest in the population, such as 'will a given intervention have an effect in a population?'. This is resolved in statistical terms by determining whether the evidence in the sample suggests that the statement 'the intervention has *no* effect in the population' is likely to be *false*. The statement is called the **null hypothesis**. So, rather than attempting to answer the original question and show that it is likely that the intervention has an effect, the statistical approach is to determine whether there is enough evidence in the sample to reject the null hypothesis that the intervention has no effect in the population. There are two possible conclusions that can be reached after the significance test has been performed. Either:

1   'On the basis of the sample, there is good evidence to suggest that the

intervention will have some effect in the population', or

2   The sample has not provided enough information to safely conclude that the statement 'the intervention has no effect in the population' is false'.

In the language of statistics, if the sample result implies that there would be an effect of the intervention in the population, the effect is said to be **statistically significant**. However, if the sample study does not provide sufficient information to reject the statement, the effect is said to 'Fail to reach statistical significance'. An effect that is statistically significant is unlikely to have arisen merely because of sampling error. Another way of explaining statistical significance is to say that there is a very small chance or *probability* of obtaining the observed results, or even more extreme results, *if the null hypothesis is true*. This probability is called the ***P*-value** of the test so that statistical significance is achieved if this *P*-value is small, typically less than the (arbitrary) cut-off value 0·05, called the **significance level**. The effect is then said to be significant at the 5% level.

It is important to distinguish between the use of the word 'significant' in statistics with its use in everyday English. Colloquially, the word 'significant' is synonymous with 'important', perhaps in some clinical or public health sense. In statistical parlance, 'significant' means 'unlikely to be caused by sampling error.' Notice that a statistically significant effect could be small and of very little clinical importance. Conversely, an observed effect may be found to be not statistically significant at the 5% level because of inadequate sample size, even though, if the intervention were applied to the population, it might have a very important clinical effect. In this context it is crucial to note that a finding of 'not significant' does not 'prove' that the intervention will have no effect in the population; it merely indicates that there is insufficient evidence to say that it will have an effect. For this and other reasons, although until relatively recently statistical results in published medical and dental papers tended to report in terms of significance levels (eg $0·01 < P < 0·05$ or $0·001 < P < 0·01$), the modern trend is to quote exact *P*-values (eg $P = 0·03$ or $P = 0·007$) and concentrate on 95% confidence intervals. Many leading journals now will not accept papers which do not follow this trend.

The next chapter will take a further look at types of study design for statistical analysis.

I   Bulman J S, Osborn J F. *Statistics in Dentistry*. London: British Dental Association, 1989.

Research designs 2

Observational versus experimental designs

Studies may be either observational or experimental. An **experimental** study is one in which the investigator deliberately intervenes so that it is possible to observe the effect of the intervention on the response of interest, usually with a view to establishing whether a change in the response is attributable to the intervention. A clinical trial is an example of an experimental study. An **observational** study is one in which the investigators do not intervene in any way, so they do not, for example, administer treatments or withhold factors which may influence the outcome of interest. An **epidemiological** study is concerned with investigating the effect of certain factors and their inter-relationships on disease. The study is usually devised with a view to eliciting possible causes of the disease, and is generally observational rather than experimental because the potential aetiological factors are often not amenable to random allocation, perhaps for ethical reasons. So, for example, in a study of the effect of cigarette smoking on the incidence of oral cancer it would be impossible (illegal and unethical) to randomly allocate individuals or communities to various levels of consumption of a potential carcinogen.

Both experimental and observational studies have much in common and it is perhaps unfortunate that some people regard the methodology of experimental research as 'medical (or dental) statistics' and the methodology of observational studies as 'surveys' or 'epidemiology'.

The effects of suspected confounding variables can be investigated in an observational study. However, if confounding variables exist without being suspected, they may misleadingly distort the apparent effect of the risk factor under study. This is the main disadvantage of an observational study; the observed effect of the factor under investigation may be due to an unsuspected confounding factor.

Observational studies

Observational studies may be **cross-sectional** or **longitudinal**. Cross-sectional studies provide a snapshot picture of a community at a point in time, and do not involve following a group of individuals over time. In contrast, **longitudinal** studies are those which require the individuals to be investigated over a period of time. The study may be **prospective** (eg a cohort study) in which case the data are collected forward in time from a given starting point. On the other hand, **retrospective** studies (eg case-control studies) are those in which the information on the individual is obtained by going backwards in time to events that have occurred, possibly relying on case records to obtain the relevant information. It should be noted that although experimental studies, by their very nature, are invariably longitudinal, observational studies may be either cross-sectional or longitudinal.

The advantages of cross-sectional studies are that they are fairly quick, easy and cheap to perform. However, they cannot provide evidence of a temporal relationship between the risk factors and disease since the data concerning exposure to the factor and the presence or absence of disease are collected simultaneously.

Sample surveys
A **sample survey** is a particular form of cross-sectional observational study in which a sample of individuals is taken from a well defined population with the intention of using the observed characteristics in the sample as estimates of the corresponding characteristics in the population. In general, the sample might be used to estimate any characteristic, but commonly the estimate would be the average value of some measurement such as age, systolic blood pressure etc or an estimate of the proportion of the individuals in a population who possess a particular attribute. If the attribute were a disease, this proportion would be called the prevalence of the disease.

Cohort studies
A cohort study (Fig. 1) involves observing and monitoring a group of individuals over a period of time. Such studies come under a number of different guises, particularly in epidemiology, with names such as *cohort* studies, *longitudinal* studies and *prospective* studies, and although these studies may involve different definitions of the study population, the statistical

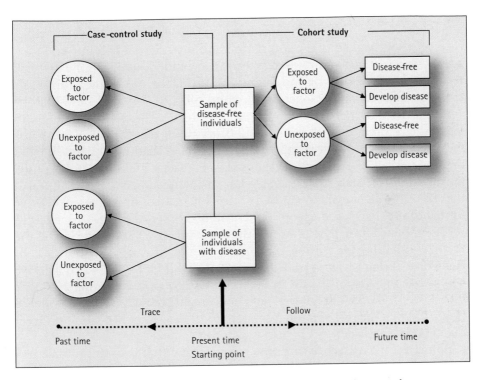

Fig. 1 Diagrammatic representation of a case-control and a cohort study.

analysis of each is essentially the same.

In a cohort study, the individuals in the sample from the relevant study population are first categorised according to the levels of the factor or factors of interest, perhaps a risk factor such as daily cigarette consumption so that each individual is classified as a current smoker or non-smoker. This cohort of individuals is then monitored for a period of time and a change in status is noted. In an epidemiological study, the status may change, for example from 'without disease' to 'with disease', where the 'disease' might be oral cancer or the loss of at least one tooth. Such changes may be measured by the rate at which new cases of the disease occur in the study population. This rate is usually called the incidence rate of the disease. The observed *incidence rates* in the risk factor categories are then compared, usually by calculating their *ratio*, called a **relative risk**.

Suppose, for example, a sample comprised 1,000 individuals aged 60+ years, each of whom had an oral examination and interview at baseline and then again 2 years later. Two hundred (20%) of the individuals lost one or more teeth during the 2 year period. Eighty (32%) of the 250 of the individuals categorised as current smokers at baseline and 120 (16%) of the 750 non-smokers lost at least one tooth in that time (Table 1). The relative risk of tooth loss is thus estimated as RR = 32/16 = 2·0, indicating that the risk of tooth loss in current smokers was twice that of non-smokers. A relative risk of one implies that the risks of disease in those exposed to the factor and those not exposed are the same. A relative risk greater (or less) than one shows the extent to which the risk of the disease in the exposed group is increased (or decreased) relative to that of the unexposed group. The confidence interval for the true relative risk is evaluated by first determining the standard error (SE) of the $\log_e$ of the relative risk, and then using the theory of the Normal distribution.[1] In particular, $SE(\log_e RR) = \sqrt{\{1/80 - 1/250 + 1/120 - 1/750\}} = 0·124$ and the 95% confidence interval for the RR in the tooth loss example is $\exp\{\log_e 2 \pm 1·96 \times 0·124\} = 1·57$ to $2·55$. This interval does not contain one and so there is evidence ($P < 0·05$) that the risk of tooth loss is significantly greater in current smokers than in non-smokers.

Sometimes, particularly for policy development, it is useful to measure how much disease burden is caused by certain modifiable risk factors. For example, the investigator may wish to answer the question 'Amongst smokers, what percentage of the total risk of tooth loss is due to smoking?' A suitable measure that provides an answer to this question involves the calculation of the **attributable risk** which is the difference between the tooth loss incidence rates in the risk factor categories.

Although a cohort study is time-consuming and costly, and is useful only for studying a common disease, it has the advantages that it can be used to study many disease outcomes as well as rare risk factors.

Table I Frequencies of individuals with some or no tooth loss in a cohort study

	Current smoker	Non-smoker	Total
Lost ≥ one tooth	80 (32%)	120 (16%)	200
Lost no teeth	170	630	800
Total	250	750	1000

Case-control studies

In a case-control study (Fig. 1), sometimes called a *case-referent, retrospective* or *trohoc* (cohort spelt backwards) study, a sample of cases, ie persons diagnosed as having the disease of interest, is compared with a group of comparable controls who do not have the disease. The cases and controls are separately categorised according to whether or not each has been exposed to the risk factor. Since it impossible to estimate the relative risk directly in a case-control study (as the relative risk requires knowledge of disease rates rather then exposure rates), it is common to estimate the **odds ratio** instead. The odds of the disease in those exposed to the factor is the chance of having the disease in those exposed to the factor divided by the chance of not having the disease in this group of individuals. The odds of disease in those not exposed to the factor is defined in a similar fashion. Then the odds ratio is the odds of disease in those exposed to the factor divided by the odds of disease in those not exposed to the factor. The odds ratio is a reasonable estimate of the relative risk of disease in those who are and are not exposed to the factor provided the disease is rare and so its prevalence is low.

Consider, for example, a case-control study which was performed to investigate the association, if any, between betel nut chewing and oral mucosal lichen lesions in women in Cambodia.[2] It was found that 5 (23·8%) of the 21 women with lichen lesions chewed betel nut, while among the 1,469 controls (ie women without lichen lesions), 127 (8.6%) chewed betel nut (Table 2). So the estimated odds of lichen lesions in those who chewed betel nut was (5/132)/(127/132) = 5/127, and the estimated odds of lichen lesions in those who did not chew betel nut was (16/1358)/(1342/1358) = 16/1342. The prevalence of lichen lesions in this group of women was low and equal to $100 \times 21/1490 = 1·4\%$. Hence, the estimated odds ratio of (5/127)/(16/1342) =

Table 2 Frequencies of women with and without lichen lesions in a case-control study			
	Women with lichen lesions	Women without lichen lesions	Total
Chewed betel nut	5 (23·8%)	127 (8·6%)	132
Did not chew betel nut	16	1342	1358
Total	21	1469	1490

$(5 \times 1342)/(127 \times 16) = 3\cdot3$ could be used to estimate the relative risk. This implies that the risk of lichen lesions was $3\cdot3$ times greater in women who chewed betel nut than in those who did not chew betel nut. A confidence interval can be determined for the true odds ratio since it can be shown that the sampling distribution of $\log_e(OR)$ approximates a Normal distribution and that $SE[\log_e(OR)] = \sqrt{(1/a + 1/b + 1/c + 1/d)}$ where a, b, c and d are the numbers of individuals exposed and not exposed to the risk factor in those with and in those without the disease. In the lichen lesion example, $\log_e(OR) = 1\cdot19$ and $SE[\log_e(OR)] = \sqrt{(1/5 + 1/16 + 1/127 + 1/1342)} = 0\cdot52$ Thus the 95% confidence interval for the logarithm of the true odds ratio is $\log_e(OR) \pm 1\cdot96 \times SE[\log_e(OR)] = 1\cdot19 \pm 1\cdot96 \times 0\cdot52 = 0\cdot173$ to $2\cdot215$. Hence the 95% confidence interval for the true odds ratio is $e^{0\cdot173}$ to $e^{2\cdot215} = 1\cdot19$ to $9\cdot16$. This confidence interval excludes one, indicating that the odds ratio is significantly different from one ($P < 0\cdot05$) and that the risk of lichen lesions in the Cambodian women from which this sample was taken was significantly greater if they chewed betel nut.

This essentially simple design can be elaborated to include stratification, matching and regression analysis to control the influence of confounding variables on the estimated relative risk. Multiple regression is discussed in greater detail in Chapter 6.

The disadvantages of a case-control study are that it is not possible to estimate the relative risk directly from the study (although if the prevalence of the disease is low, the odds ratio can be used as an estimate of the relative risk), that selection of the controls may be difficult and that it is possible to study only a single disease outcome in any one study. However, case-control studies are relatively quick, easy and cheap to perform, and can be used to study many risk factors as well as rare diseases.

Experimental studies

If the study is experimental rather than observational then it must be designed in such a way that it gains the largest amount of information of the greatest reliability in an efficient manner. The objective, therefore, is to achieve an optimal balance between minimal sample size and maximum precision whilst eliminating sources of bias and identifying and controlling all sources of variation. This balance may be achieved by choosing the appropriate experimental design which takes into account the particular circumstances of the investigation.

Invariably, a well-designed experiment is both **comparative** and **randomised**. The comparison is usually between the unauthenticated novel intervention (such as a treatment or preventative measure) and some form of 'control', such as an established intervention. Randomisation, also called random allocation, implies that the subjects are randomly (ie using a method based on chance) assigned the treatments or interventions. One advantage of randomisation is that potential confounding factors will be approximately evenly distributed in the different intervention groups. So, for example, in a study of the effects of a therapeutic dentifrice in the treatment of periodontal conditions in a large multiracial society, random allocation of the subjects to the dentifrice or control 'treatments' would ensure that each ethnic group is approximately equally represented in both the study and control groups. This would be important if ethnic group were associated both with the use of the dentifrice and the periodontal condition, with consequent difficulties in separating the effects of these factors on the outcome.

The **clinical trial**[3] is a particular form of experimental study which is afforded special consideration because the experiment is performed on humans. Particular attention must be focused on the ethical problems that arise in medical and dental research. Designing the trial so as to use the minimum number of patients enabling a valid conclusion regarding the efficacy of treatments to be drawn must be a major objective in the clinical scenario. A full discussion of the clinical trial, randomisation and sample size calculations is given in Chapters 3 and 4.

One important distinguishing feature of any experimental design is whether the treatment comparisons are made *between* subjects (parallel groups designs) or *within* subjects (matched designs or cross-over studies).

Parallel groups
Parallel groups designs involve the basic observational units (typically, the subjects) being independently and randomly allocated to two or more treatment groups. The response is observed for every individual in the study and an aggregate measure (usually an arithmetic mean or median if the response is quantitative or a proportion if the response is qualitative) is calculated for each treatment group. These summary measures are then compared appropriately so that the investigator can determine whether the responses differ significantly in the different treatment groups. The parallel groups design therefore relies on comparisons which are made between groups

of subjects. It should be noted that although generally desirable, it is not necessary to have an equal number of subjects in each group.

If there are two treatment groups and the response is quantitative and satisfies the assumptions underlying the method, the comparison of response to treatments may be afforded by the two-sample *t*-test. If there are more than two treatment groups, the one-way analysis of variance facilitates treatment comparisons, provided the assumptions underlying the method are satisfied. If the response is qualitative, the chi-square test is often employed for comparative purposes.

The randomised parallel groups design has the advantages that it is conceptually simple and the analysis is straightforward. In some circumstances, however, it may be appropriate to modify the simple parallel groups design by employing a technique called **blocking** or **stratification** in addition to the simple randomisation of subjects to treatments. This involves forming subgroups of individuals, the blocks or strata, such that the variation with respect to the variable of interest within each stratum is smaller than the variation between the strata. Consider, for example, an analysis of the variable DMF which is higher in older children than in younger children. It may therefore lead to greater precision for a given total sample size (or alternatively equal precision for a smaller sample size) if the overall group of children is stratified by age, and the older age-group analysed separately from the younger. In other words, the individuals are randomly allocated to the different treatments in each age stratum so that a simple parallel groups design is contained within each of these age strata. Subsequent treatment comparisons are made between groups of subjects within each stratum, and the results properly combined to determine the overall treatment effect.

Stratification may also be employed because it is of interest to investigate whether the effect of treatment (say the difference in response in the two or more treatment groups) is the same for all strata of the study population. For example, is the effect of treatment the same for younger children as it is for older children? If the treatment effect depends on the factor defining the blocks or strata, there is an interaction between the treatment and the factor. This would clearly be important for identifying patients who would benefit from a new treatment.

Even if the effect of the treatment or intervention were the same at every level of the blocked or stratified factor, the response might change systematically with the factor. For example, the average effect of the treatment (that is, the difference between the average responses to two treatments), may be the same in every age group, but the response may tend to increase with age. By making the comparison between the two treatment groups within each age group, the factor age will not confound the treatment effect. Furthermore, by controlling the potential confounding effect of a variable such as age, the precision of the comparison between the two groups will be improved.

Thus the advantages of blocking or stratifying the study population before randomisation are to enable interactions to be detected and estimated, to control the effect of known potential confounding factors and to improve precision. The disadvantage is that the statistical analysis is slightly more complicated.

Matched designs

If the blocking described above is carried to extremes, then pairs of subjects (or triplets if there are three treatment categories) can be matched so that they are alike with respect to a number of potential confounding factors. For example, if it were decided to match for age and sex, the subjects in the study would be arranged in pairs so that the two individuals in each pair would be the same age and sex. The two individual subjects in each matched pair would then be randomly allocated to different treatment/intervention groups. The comparison between the two treatments is made within each matched pair and thus the treatment effect will be more precisely estimated than it would be with a parallel groups study with the same number of subjects.

The analysis of matched studies is relatively straightforward and is often achieved by using the paired t-test for matched quantitative data or, if the data are dichotomous, McNemar's test.

The advantage of a matched study compared with a parallel groups design is a gain in precision with the same number of subjects, or equivalently, the same degree of precision of a parallel groups study can be achieved with a smaller total number of subjects.

The disadvantages of matching are that the study may become logistically difficult if too many matching factors are included and the inability to match some subjects may reduce the total number of subjects in the study. It may be more difficult to investigate interactions in a matched study.

Cross-over trials

The matched pairs study enables treatment comparisons to be made using similar experimental units. Rather than these experimental units being different subjects who have been matched appropriately, a similar type of study is one in which the subject acts as his/her own control with the same subject being allocated both treatments, receiving them at different times. Such designs are called cross-over designs[4] because the subject crosses over from one treatment to the other. The designs should involve randomising the order of administration of the treatments to each subject. The treatment comparison is then made within subjects and, in the same way as a matched pairs study, increases the precision of the treatment effect for a given number of subjects.

Designs in which the subject receives both treatments are sometimes regarded as an extreme form of matching. However, the difference between extreme matching and using the subject as her/his own control arises because with matched pairs the subjects are randomly allocated to treatments, whereas in the cross-over trial the subject acts as his own control and thus receives both treatments. In the analysis of simple studies, this difference may not matter but with more complicated designs the fact that the main observational unit, the subject, is split between the two treatments may need to be taken into account.

Cross-over trials, although advantageous when compared to parallel groups designs in terms of precision or sample size, cannot be utilized for conditions which do not remain stable in the study period or which can be cured by the treatments being administered, when there is a carry-over effect from one treatment to another, or when the response to treatment is prolonged.

The choice of observational unit

A fundamental consideration in research designs concerns the choice of observational unit.[5] It is important to understand that the unit of observation in an experiment or observational study is the smallest unit with a unique set of important characteristics which is independent of other similar units in that its response cannot be affected by these other units, and which can be assigned to each of the treatments in an experimental study. Thus the observational or experimental unit in a clinical trial is often the patient or, in the case of dental investigations, the mouth because teeth cannot be regarded as independent units within the mouth. The experiment should be designed and analysed with this in mind so, for example, the randomisation process should randomise the mouths (the experimental units) rather than the teeth (the sub-units) to the different treatments. In the same way, the sample size estimation process whilst satisfying certain criteria, must aim to estimate the optimal number of experimental units rather than the sub-units contained within them.[6]

As an example, consider just two situations where either the individual child or a 'community' of children, say a school, is the basic unit of observation. For example, in a randomised intervention study of fluoride supplement, if the individual child was the basic unit, individual children would be randomly allocated to receive the intervention or not, whereas if the basic unit was the school, then the schools would be randomly allocated and the responses would be observed for individual children within their school. The difference between these two types of design is very important. An extreme example may make this clearer. Suppose 1,000 children attend ten schools and it is of interest to investigate the effect of fluoride supplementation on DMF. Two designs that might be considered are:

1 Take each child and randomly allocate it either to receive the supplement, or not, and after 1 year compare the means of the changes in DMF in the two groups of 500 children.

2 Give the supplement to all the children in five randomly chosen schools and withhold it from all the children in the other schools. Calculate the mean change in DMF in each school and then compare the means of these mean changes in the two groups of five schools.

Clearly, in Design 1, where the individual child is the basic unit, a more precise estimate of the effect of supplementation (ie one with a narrower confidence interval) will be obtained than in Design 2 where the comparison may be confounded by other differences between the schools. Design 2 could be improved if there were many more schools available for randomisation.

The advantages and disadvantages of the two designs are:

1 For a given total number of children, studies with the child as the basic unit will be more precise and have a greater power to detect an effect of treatment than if the schools are the observational units.

2 Equivalently, to achieve a given level of precision, more children are required for a school based study than if the children themselves are the observational units. This increase in sample size (or loss of precision) is often called the *design effect* of the study.

3 Logistically, it is often much easier to organise and administer a study based on schools rather than children. In extreme cases, for example a

community intervention such as the introduction of piped water, it may be impossible to conduct a study based on individual persons.

4 For a given total monetary budget (including the costs of all resources used, such as manpower, equipment, travel etc), it will usually be possible to have a larger total sample size if schools are the observational units. This increase in sample size will sometimes more than offset the advantages, discussed in Points 1 and 2, of studies with child based units.

5 Analysis is usually easier if a study is based on independent individuals rather than schools, but clearly the availability of computers and user-friendly packages for statistical analysis makes this advantage less important.

In a sample survey, the simplest design in which the observational unit (for example, a village) comprises a collection of individual units (for example, people) leads to a *cluster* analysis.[7] The clusters (the villages) are randomly selected and all the individual units (people) within each selected cluster are observed. This design may be extended to multi-stage or hierarchical sampling.

In an experimental study, the design in which the main experimental units (for example, mouths) containing sub-units (for example, teeth) are assigned to different treatments leads to a *split-plot, split-unit, nested,*[8] *multi-level* or *hierarchical*[9] analysis. The difficulty with analysing such designs is that there are two sources of sampling error: that arising from the differences between sub-units units within each main unit and that caused by differences between main units. In almost all situations, the contribution of the differences between main units to the overall sampling error will be much greater than that contributed by sub-units within each main unit. It can be shown that for a fixed total study size, it is desirable (but more costly) to have a large number of main units and to observe fewer sub-units in each main unit. This same problem arises in clinical trials in which repeated observations are made on each subject. An example of such a clinical trial is a study of gingivitis (inflammation of the gums) in which there are three treatments, a variable number of patients in each treatment group and a variable number of sites where the gums are inflamed within each patient's mouth. The main units are the patients and the sub-units are the sites. Some aspects of the problem of the choice of units to use for the statistical analysis are considered in Chapter 7 on repeated measures.

1 Altman D G. *Practical Statistics for Medical Research*. UK: CRC press, 1991.
2 Ikeda N, Handa Y, Khim S P, Durward C, Axell T, Mizuna T, Fukano H, Kawai T. Prevalence study of oral mucosal lesions in a selected Cambodian population. *Community Dent Oral Epidemiol* 1995; 2 3: 49-54.
3 Pocock S J. *Clinical Trials: a Practical Approach*. Chichester: Wiley, 1983 .
4 Senn S. *Cross-Over Trials in Clinical Research*. Chichester: Wiley, 1993.
5 Altman D G, Bland J M. Units of analysis. *Br Med J* 1997; 3 1 4: 1874.
6 Kerry S M, Bland J M. Sample size in cluster randomisation. *Br Med J* 1998; 3 1 6: 549.
7 Cochran W G. *Sampling Techniques*. 3rd edn. Wiley: New York, 1977.
8 Scheffé H. *The Analysis of Variance*. New York: Wiley, 1999.
9 Sullivan L S, Dukes K A, Losina E. An introduction to hierarchical linear modelling. *Stat Med* 1999; 1 8: 855-888.

Clinical trials 1

The **clinical trial** is a planned experiment, strictly on human subjects, which is conducted with a view to investigating the efficacy of one or more treatments for a given condition. It is possible to use statistical techniques to make inferences about the population of patients who will present to the practitioner in the future using information obtained from the sample of patients in the trial. Consequently, the results of the trial may be expected to influence the way in which patients with the condition are treated in the future.

This chapter discusses some of the more important design and analysis considerations underlying clinical trials. In particular, the comparative nature of clinical trials, the need for randomisation and blinding techniques, the ethical problems inherent in 'experimenting' on human subjects and analysis by intention-to-treat are discussed in some depth. Chapter 4 concentrates on sample size estimation with some discussion of sequential and interim analyses. More details of all aspects of clinical trials can be obtained from Pocock,[1] whilst the considerations which govern the quality of reporting of clinical trials are described in the CONSORT statement (www.consort-statement.org).

Trial design

It is crucial that the clinical trial be designed and analysed so that its results are unbiased and any conclusions drawn from it are valid. Bias is present when the trial results are systematically distorted and so are consistently above (or below) what they should be. Various sources of bias were briefly discussed in Chapter 1(Research Designs 1). Design considerations are particularly important because, although it is possible to correct an inappropriate analysis or weak presentation, it is often impossible to rectify the situation once the data have been collected in a trial which has deficiencies in design. A well-designed trial is one which, at the very least, is comparative in nature and incorporates randomisation of patients to treatments; it is then called a **randomised controlled trial** (RCT).

Use of a 'control' treatment

An essential feature of a clinical trial is that it is *comparative* in nature. This means that it is necessary to compare the results of a group of patients who are receiving the new treatment under investigation with another group of similar patients under some different treatment regime. This other treatment regime, the **control** treatment, may be an active treatment (a *positive* control) such as a standard treatment that has been shown previously to be effective. Alternatively, if ethical considerations permit, the other treatment regime may be the absence of active treatment or else a dummy treatment, called a **placebo**, both of which are *negative* controls. A placebo is an inert substance which looks just like the active treatment. Its purpose is to separate the act of being treated from the real effect of the active treatment. Many individuals are influenced by suggestion and respond to the act of receiving treatment, producing what is often called the 'placebo-effect'.

A clinical trial which includes a comparative group is called a **controlled** clinical trial. The reason for making the trial controlled is to ensure that, provided the composition of the treatment groups is similar, any conclusions drawn from the trial as to the effectiveness of the new treatment under consideration can be attributed solely to the administration of that treatment and not to any other factors.

There are some researchers who advocate the use of **historical controls** instead of or, sometimes, in addition to concurrent controls. Historical controls are individuals who have received the standard treatment in a previous trial so that the results of the current patients on the new treatment under investigation can be compared to these historical controls. This obviates the need for randomisation as all patients in the trial can be assigned to the new treatment.

Some researchers prefer this retrospective approach for two reasons. Firstly, fewer patients are required in the current trial. Secondly, it overcomes the ethical problem the practitioner faces when obliged to put as many patients on the standard treatment as on the new treatment which the practitioner believes (intuitively) to be superior. Similarly, the patients may well have convictions about the advantages of the new treatment, and they will only consent to being included in a trial which ensures that this is what they will receive. However, there is always the danger that the results from the historical controls are not strictly comparable to those of the current patients. This may be a consequence of differences in the type of patient, the severity of the illness, the ancillary treatment, the criteria for evaluating response, the quality of recorded data and the intensity of monitoring of the patients. The overall effect of such a retrospective comparison is that the efficacy of the new treatment is usually overestimated which leads to a biased result. The controversy rages on but the policy of not using historical controls, except in the situation in which the condition is rare and there are few patients available for the trial, is invariably promoted.

Randomisation
It may be that the clinician has a preconceived notion as to the effectiveness of the new treatment and this will influence the way in which the patients are allocated to various treatments, if given the freedom of choice. This might result in the more severely ill patients being allocated the standard treatment, or *vice-versa*, even if the clinician's intention is to be fair, and this in turn would result in a biased estimate of the treatment effect. In order to avoid the possibility of this happening, the patients are *randomly* assigned treatments. This means that the method of determining which treatment each patient receives relies on chance rather than on personal judgement so that the potential for allocation bias is obviated.

Random allocation (ie randomisation) can be achieved by some mechanical method such as tossing a coin, but is more usually accomplished by using random number tables or computer generated random numbers. To illustrate randomisation, consider a trial in which there are two treatments, A and B, for a given condition. One 'random number' approach to allocating a patient one of the two treatments is to refer to a random number table (found in many statistical texts as well as in books of statistical tables). The table consists quite simply of blocks of the digits 0–9 which have been generated in a random manner. Each block usually consists of five numbers by five, for example:

69373
95662
97758
12154
25583

A complete table, with all digits equally represented, will consist of a grid of these blocks. To use the table, a starting point is selected at random, and then the sequence of digits is followed along a row or up or down a column. Suppose that the starting point is the top left hand '6' in the above section of the table, and the decision has been made previously to follow the sequence

25

down the columns, and to allocate the next patient presenting to the clinic to 'A' if the digit is even, and to 'B' if the digit is odd (including zeros which are regarded as even). Thus the sequence 6, 9, 9, 1 and 2 would result in the first five patients successively receiving A, B, B, B and A. Starting at the top of the next column, the sequence 9, 5, 7, 2 and 5 would result in the next five patients successively receiving B, B, B, A and B; and so on. It can be seen, in this particular allocation sequence, that if the trial consisted only of 10 patients, three patients would be allocated to 'A' and seven patients would be allocated to 'B'. Such an imbalance is undesirable and yet is not uncommon if the sample size is small.

Fortunately, the simple random allocation procedure can be modified, for example, to allow each patient to be allocated one of three or more treatments, or, using a process called **balanced** or **blocked randomisation**, to achieve approximately equal numbers of patients in the different treatments groups. Suppose two treatments, A and B, are to be compared, and it is decided that balance is required after every group or block of k patients, where k is some multiple of two (the number of treatments). For illustrative purposes, let $k = 8$. Using the randomisation technique described in the previous paragraph on the first block of 8 patients, each successive patient is randomly allocated either A or B depending on whether the next random number in the sequence is odd or even. However, as soon as $k/2 = 4$ patients have been allocated one treatment, say A, the remaining patients in the group of 8 patients who have not yet been allocated a treatment have to be allocated the other treatment, B. This will result in 4 patients in each treatment group in the first block of 8 patients. If this process is repeated for the next block of 8 patients, then of the 16 patients in the two blocks, 8 patients will be in each treatment group. If this process is repeated a number of times, exactly half the patients will receive A and the other half will receive B if the total sample size is a multiple of 8. If the total sample size is not a multiple of 8, then approximately half the patients will be in each treatment group, and this is usually satisfactory for purposes of analysis.

Clearly, randomisation promotes comparability of the treatment groups with respect to the effects of extraneous variables which might influence the response to treatment, such as the age or sex of the patient or the severity of the disease. Although the researchers may believe they are aware of which variables are likely to influence response, and may attempt to ensure that the treatment groups are similar with respect to these variables (using *stratified* randomization), it may be that there are other relevant extraneous variables about whose effects they are unaware. By randomising the patients to the different treatments, it is possible to ensure that the treatment groups are balanced, on average, for all extraneous variables of consequence.

Two factors should be noted in relation to randomisation. Firstly, *randomisation* (or *random allocation*) should be distinguished from *random sampling*.[2] The former is concerned with deciding which patients should receive the different treatments. The latter is concerned with deciding which patients to select from the population for inclusion in the trial. In randomisation, the patients are *given* treatments; in random sampling, the patients are *taken* from the population. Both, however, rely on chance to achieve their ends. Secondly, it can be shown that random allocation obviates the need for strict random sampling from larger populations, one of the assumptions underlying statistical hypothesis testing which is an important component in the analysis of clinical trials.

Blinding

Another source of potential bias arises from the assessment of the response to treatment. Both the patient receiving treatment and the assessor of the response to treatment may have preconceived notions about the superiority of one treatment over another. If either was aware of which treatment the patient was receiving, this might influence the assessor's assessment of response and lead to a biased result. Such a biased assessment may be intentional or, more usually, subconscious or unintentional, and is more likely to occur when the response to treatment is subjective rather than objective.

One way of controlling this assessment bias is to conduct the trial in such a way that the clinician, the support staff, the patient and the assessor of the response to treatment are unaware of which treatment the patient is receiving. Such a trial is called a **double-blind trial**. In order to make the trial double-blind, it is important that the treatments that are being compared look, taste and feel identical. If one of the treatments is a non-active control treatment, this can only be achieved by introducing a dummy or placebo as the negative control. If the form of administration of the different treatments differ, for example if one treatment comprises a toothpaste and a second treatment comprises a mouthwash, then it is possible to make the treatments appear identical by having one group receive the active toothpaste with a dummy mouthwash and the other group receive the dummy toothpaste with an active mouthwash.

It is not always possible, either because of ethical considerations or because of practical difficulties, to make the trial double-blind. For example, it would hardly be ethical to mimic an invasive procedure such as surgery in order to facilitate blindness, and it would be impossible for a surgeon to be blind to the particular treatment that a patient is receiving. In such circumstances, the aim should be to make the trial **single-blind** so that the assessor of the response to treatment is unaware of the treatment that the patient has received. If the response to treatment is objective rather than subjective in nature, then concerns regarding assessment bias, provided that the trial is at least single-blind, are substantially alleviated.

Ethical problems

The most serious objection to randomised controlled trials arises because of the ethical dilemma facing the researcher. There is a conflict between what might be termed *individual* and *collective* ethics. On the one hand, the practitioner would like to administer the treatment which is regarded as most beneficial for the particular patient; on the other hand, he or she is attempting to evaluate different treatments with a view to establishing, for a future population of hypothetical patients, the most effective treatment for a given condition.

There is no easy solution to this ethical dilemma. A balance has to be struck between concern for the individual and human experimentation for the advancement of science. At no stage should the former be sacrificed for the latter. To achieve this balance, it is important to employ safeguards for the individual patient and also to design and conduct the trial so that high scientific and organisational standards are attained throughout.

Guidelines for the ethical requirements of clinical research are outlined in the World Medical Association Declaration of Helsinki: Recommendations Guiding Medical Doctors in Biomedical Research Involving Human Subjects which was adopted in Finland in 1964 and revised most recently in Edinburgh, Scotland, in 2000. Details may be found at www.wma.net/e/policy/17-c_e.html. These guide-lines provide a basis for 'protecting' the individual. Included in them is a requirement that 'informed consent' is obtained from every patient (or legal guardian, if necessary) to be included in the trial. Informed consent implies that the patient is aware of and understands all the implications involved in the study which are known to the researchers, and is willing to accept these as a condition of his/her involvement in the study. An additional safeguard adopted in the UK is the requirement that all proposals come before local ethical committees whose members, comprising both lay individuals and clinicians, discuss the ethical implications of the proposed trial.

All aspects of the trial, including its rationale, patient selection criteria, treatment schedules and methods of evaluation, design, study size, proposed statistical analysis, patient consent, forms, withdrawals and administrative responsibilities, must be specified in a document called a **protocol**. The protocol is produced before the trial is undertaken. It ensures that all relevant and important considerations which lead to a scientifically worthwhile study are considered at the outset whilst, at the same time, an indication is given of the procedure to be adopted for each individual patient.

Intention-to-treat analysis

One of the major difficulties when analysing clinical trials is knowing how best to handle what are termed **protocol violations**. These are patients who fail, for any one of a number of reasons, to complete the intended course of treatment; they are called **withdrawals**.

Sometimes a withdrawal results in there being incomplete data for evaluation for that patient, and it is unrelated to the condition or treatment of the patient. It may be that the patient fails to turn up to the clinic because of moving out of the area or simply because the patient is tired of the commitment. Alternatively, the incomplete information may be caused by administrative errors so that some measurements are missing. One has to hope that the number of missing observations is not too great in these circumstances, establish that their omission does not create any biases, and then analyse the data without them.

From time to time, however, a protocol violation occurs when a patient is evaluated through the length of the trial but that patient is no longer receiving the treatment that was originally assigned. For example, the patient may be switched to the alternative treatment because of side-effects or may get bored with taking a prescribed medication in a trial for a non-acute condition over a prolonged period of investigation. These protocol violations are also called withdrawals and one has to decide how best to deal with them. Should the results from these withdrawals be analysed according to what should have happened to the patients or to what actually happened to them or should they be omitted?

Although it may at first appear to go against the grain, the approach generally adopted is, wherever possible, to include all withdrawals in the statistical analysis, and analyse the results for these patients as if they were still in the treatment groups to which they were originally assigned. This approach is termed **analysis by intention-to-treat.** The rationalisation for this type of analysis is that it avoids the biases that would be introduced by the alternatives of either omitting the results or analysing the results according to the treatments that these patients actually received. Such biases could arise if the comparison groups were no longer comparable with respect to any variables likely to affect the measure of response, or if withdrawals exacerbated the efficacy of a particular treatment by excluding patients who suffered ill-effects from that treatment.

The intention-to-treat approach to analysing the results of clinical trials is often called the **pragmatic approach** because its aim is to make inferences about the effectiveness of a particular treatment regime as it is adopted in practice. The alternative **explanatory approach,** that of analysing the results only for the compliers who conform to the protocol specification, is very occasionally adopted but the aim, then, is geared to understanding the processes involved rather than to making decisions about how to treat future patients. A fuller discussion may be obtained from Schwartz, Flamart and Lellouch.[3]

1. Pocock S J. *Clinical Trials: a practical approach.* Chichester and New York: John Wiley and Sons, 1983.
2. Kish L. *Survey Sampling.* New York, John Wiley and Sons, 1995.
3. Schwartz D, Flamart R, Lellouch J. *Clinical Trials.* London: Academic Press, 1980.

Clinical trials 2

4

The principles which underlie a well-designed clinical trial were introduced in Chapter 3. The trial should be controlled (to ensure that the appropriate comparisons are made), *randomised* (to avoid allocation bias) and, preferably, *blinded* (to obviate assessment bias). However, taken in isolation, these concepts will not necessarily ensure that meaningful conclusions can be drawn from the study. It is essential that the sample size is large enough to enable the effects of interest to be estimated precisely, and to detect any real treatment differences.

Sample size estimation

'How large a sample do I need?' is one of the most commonly asked questions of a statistician. It is also one of the hardest questions to answer. The researcher posing the query usually believes, quite wrongly, that the statistician can produce a figure, as if by magic, without any information about the why's and wherefore's of the trial. Unfortunately, both life and sample size estimation are not so simple! It is necessary to have some idea of the results that are expected from the trial, *before it has been conducted*, in order to evaluate the actual sample size required. If the proposed sample size appears outrageous, it is important to realise that if the numbers are reduced substantially, it may not be possible to detect real treatment differences, even if they exist. At the other extreme, if more patients than are really needed to compare treatments are used, the study may fall short of the ethical prerequisites.

Type I and Type II errors

The fundamental ideas of sample size estimation are perhaps most easily understood in the context of a trial to compare two arithmetic means using independent samples. The null hypothesis is that the true means in the populations from which the samples are derived are equal. An example is a clinical trial to compare the cariostatic action of two toothpastes in children of a given age; the children are to be randomly allocated the toothpastes and the

Table I Errors in testing the null hypothesis, H_0

	H_0 rejected	H_0 not rejected
H_0 false	No error	Type II error
H_0 true	Type I error	No error

mean dmfs increment observed after, say, 2 years will be compared in the two groups. Alternatively, a study might be designed to investigate whether the presence of fillings affects the level of *Streptococcus mutans* in the saliva; children recruited to the study will be divided into two groups not randomly, but according to the presence or absence of fillings, and the mean level of *S. mutans* observed in samples of saliva taken from the children will be compared. At the design stage of studies such as these, it will be necessary to know how many children to include in each sample.

The decision whether or not to reject the null hypothesis depends on the magnitude of the *P*-value obtained from the test and the cut-off value for it which determines significance, ie the **significance level**. Very often, although not necessarily, this level is chosen to be 0·05 so that the null hypothesis is rejected if the *P*-value is less than 0·05. If this is so, the result is said to be statistically significant and it is concluded that there is enough evidence to reject the null hypothesis. In the examples quoted, this would imply that there is evidence to suggest that one of the toothpastes is, on average, more cariostatic than the other, or that, on average, children with fillings tend to have higher (or lower) levels of *S. mutans* than children without fillings. Alternatively, if the *P*-value is greater than the cut-off level, there is not enough evidence to reject the null hypothesis, and the observed difference between the sample means is said to be not statistically significant at the chosen level. Note, however, that this does not necessarily imply that the means in the populations of children are equal, only that there is insufficient evidence to show that that these means are different.

It must be recognised that coming to either of these conclusions may or may not be correct. Rejecting the null hypothesis when it is true (concluding that there is evidence to show that the population means differ when, in fact, they are equal) leads to what is termed a **Type I error**. A **Type II error** is made when the null hypothesis is not rejected when it is false, ie when it is concluded that there is insufficient evidence to show that the population means differ when, in fact, these means are not equal. Table 1 summarises the consequences of rejecting and not rejecting the null hypothesis in the circumstances in which it is either true or false.

Clearly both Type I and Type II errors are undesirable but because they arise as a consequence of sampling, and thus not having all information from the population available, the chances of making these errors cannot be entirely eliminated. The chances (ie probabilities) of making the Type I and Type II errors are usually denoted by the Greek letters, alpha (α) and beta (β), respectively. The aim in designing a study is to control α and β so that they are acceptable in the context of the proposed study. Since they both increase as the sample size of the study decreases, all other relevant factors remaining constant, choosing the optimal sample size becomes an integral part of study design.

The first step is to decide, in advance of collecting the data, on the worst case scenario for a Type I error. This means choosing the significance level of the test, the maximum value of α, and this is commonly but not necessarily assigned the value 0·05. Then the probability of incorrectly rejecting the null hypothesis cannot exceed 0·05 since H_0 is not rejected if $P > 0·05$. Now, if β is the probability of *not* rejecting the null hypothesis when it is false, then $(1-\beta)$ is the probability of rejecting it when it is false. $(1-\beta)$ is called the **power** of the test; it is the probability (often expressed as a percentage) of *correctly* concluding that a treatment difference of a specified size exists. It is usual to ensure that the study has a high power, very often in excess of 80%, since there is no justification for embarking on a study if it is known in advance that the study has little chance of detecting a real treatment effect. Having decided on values for the significance level and the power of the test, both of which will be chosen according to the circumstances of the investigation and the null hypothesis under test, it is then possible to evaluate the optimal sample size. However, as indicated in the following section, other factors apart from the power and the significance level come into play in the sample size determination.

Altman's nomogram

There are various approaches one can use to determine the optimal sample size, each incorporating the same relevant factors into the calculations. It is usually the specification of these factors, provided in the bullet points in the following subsections, which creates the greatest difficulty in sample size calculations. Computer programs are available, for example *nQueryAdvisor*,[1] which produce useful tables and graphs. Specific formulae

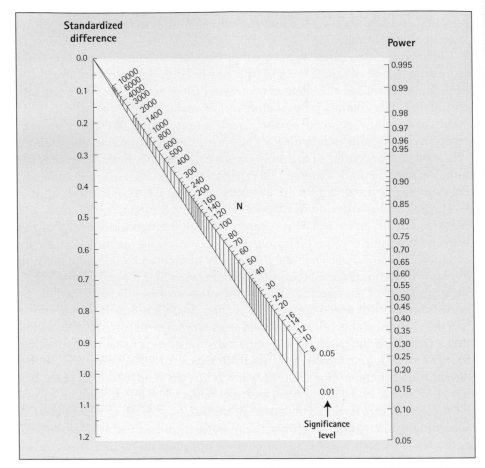

Fig. 1 Altman's nomogram for the calculation of sample size or power (extracted from Altman, 1982 How large a sample? in *Statistics in Practice*. Eds S. M. Gore and D. G. Altman. BMA London. Copyright BMJ Publishing Group, with permission).

can be used to test different hypotheses, but these formulae tend to be cumbersome and their use time-consuming. Special tables exist for sample size calculations (Machin *et al.*, 1997)[2] but the disadvantage to this approach is the need for a separate table for each type of hypothesis. An alternative, and relatively simple approach (Altman, 1982),[3] is to use the nomogram shown in Figure 1.

34

The right-hand vertical axis of the nomogram represents different power values, ranging from 0·05 to 0·995. The left-hand vertical axis represents what is termed the standardized difference. This is a ratio which relates the difference of interest to the standard deviation of the observations. The exact form of the standardized difference varies according to the nature of the variable under investigation and the specific hypothesis test. There are two axes within the nomogram, one for a significance level of 0·05, the other for 0·01, with total sample sizes indicated on each. The nomogram can be used to evaluate the optimal sample size once the power is specified, the significance level is chosen, and the standardized difference is calculated. Alternatively, the procedure can be reversed, and the power of the study determined for a specified sample size. The nomogram is used under the assumption that equal sized samples are required, but the procedure can be modified to accommodate unequal sample sizes.

Sample size calculations for the comparison of two means from independent samples

Suppose that Altman's nomogram is to be used to estimate the optimal sample size for a trial in which the mean values of a single continuous variable using independent samples are to be compared. Typically, the data would be analysed by performing a *two sample t-test*, provided the data in each group are approximately Normally distributed and the observations in the two groups are *homoscedastic* (have the same variance). But first, it would be necessary to decide how many observations to include in each sample. Suppose it were decided to have equal sample sizes (n) in each group, with a total of $N = 2n$ observations.

In order to use the nomogram, the following factors must be specified:

- The **significance level** of the test: it is usually fixed at 0·05 or, occasionally, at 0·01, and a two-sided test adopted.

- The **power** of the test: this is usually required to be of the order of 80–90%.

- The assumed constant **variance** (σ^2), of the observations in each group. Inevitably, it is difficult to specify the variance of the observations before the data have been collected. However, since the variability of the observations has a direct bearing on sample size, some estimate of it must

35

be obtained. The more variable the data, the larger the samples that are required to detect a real treatment difference of a specified size, if all other factors remain constant. It may be that a rough estimate of σ^2 can be obtained using the variance of the observations from a past experiment that has been performed which is similar in nature to that which is now planned. Perhaps the information can be found from published papers. If all else fails, it may be necessary to resort to a *pilot study* which is a small investigation, a small 'dress rehearsal' of the planned study, which may be used to provide an estimate of the variance.

- **The clinically important difference in the mean responses** (δ) which is considered to be so clinically or biologically important that if it were really to exist, it should be detectable by the proposed study. This is not the same as the difference in the mean responses which will be observed. It is a quantity that the investigator, not the statistician, must specify when he or she gives consideration to the consequences which may arise from the investigation. Note that it is easier to detect a large difference than a small one, so that the sample size is inversely proportional to δ.

In this particular problem of determining the optimal sample size to compare two means using the two sample t-test, the **standardized difference** is δ/σ, the clinically important difference divided by the assumed equal standard deviation of the observations in each group. This is the quantity on the left-hand vertical axis of the nomogram.

So, taking the first example in which two toothpastes are to be compared, suppose the investigator argues that if one toothpaste were to reduce the mean dmfs increment by 0·5 compared with the other, this would be regarded as a worthwhile treatment difference. There is an implication that if the true difference were less than 0·5, the investigator would not be too disappointed if the result was not statistically significant. The investigator must also obtain an estimate of the standard deviation, σ, of the dmfs increments. Researching the literature for other studies of the progression of dental caries in children, one obtains an estimate of the standard deviation, say $\sigma = 1·25$ dmfs increment. Then the standardized difference is $\delta/\sigma = 0·5/1·25 = 0·4$. If the investigator specifies that the level of significance to be adopted for the two-sided test is 0·05 and that the power should be 90% (often a rather arbitrary decision), the nomogram can be used to determine the total number of children required in the study. The line produced by connecting (using a ruler) the value of 0·4 for

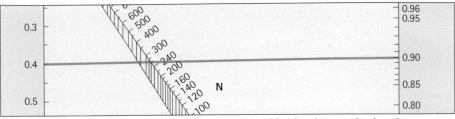

Fig. 2 The line produced by connecting the value of 0·4 for the standardized difference to the power value of 0·90 cuts the axis for a significance level of 0·05 at about N = 260 (a magnified section of Fig. I is shown)

the standardized difference to the power value of 0·90 cuts the axis for a significance level of 0·05 at about $N = 260$ (Fig. 2). This indicates that there should be approximately $n = 130$ children in each toothpaste group. The investigator should then include in the protocol, paper or grant application a power statement such as 'it was decided to have 130 children in each of the two toothpaste groups in order to have a 90% chance of detecting a difference in mean dmfs increments of 0.5 at the 5% level of significance, assuming the standard deviation of dmfs increments to be about 1·25 in each of the groups'.

It must be remembered that a sample size calculation can never be totally precise since the quantities used to calculate the sample size are often guessed or imprecisely estimated. The aim of the calculation is to obtain a 'ball-park' figure for the sample size that is practically viable and results in a test which has sufficient power to detect a real and important treatment difference. The appeal of the nomogram is that it is easy to repeat the calculations after altering one or more of the quantities required to estimate the sample size. This is not to say it should be used deviously or to 'fiddle the figures'. As an illustration, suppose the sample size of 260 in the example quoted is unrealistic. What will be the effect on sample size of reducing the power specification from 90% to 80%? Again, using a ruler to connect the appropriate numbers in the nomogram, it can be seen that this would reduce the total sample size from 260 to about 200 (Fig. 3).

Sample size calculations for other comparisons

The use of the nomogram is fairly straightforward when it is necessary to compare two means from independent groups. The principles underlying the use of the nomogram remain the same for other types of experiment; essentially, it is the form of the standardized difference which changes. The

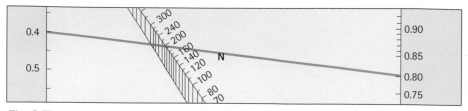

Fig. 3 The line produced by connecting the value of 0·4 for the standardized difference to the power value of 0·80 cuts the axis for a significance level of 0·05 at about $N = 200$ (a magnified section of Fig. 1 is shown)

two sided significance level (usually 0·05) and the power, usually between 80% and 90%, must still be specified for these calculations. The standardized differences that are required for different comparisons are indicated in the following bullet points.

- *Comparing two groups of paired numerical data* . The paired *t*-test is used to test the null hypothesis that the mean difference of a quantitative variable in two dependent or paired groups is zero. The standardized difference is

$$2\delta/\sigma_d$$

 where:

 δ is the clinically important difference.

 σ_d is the standard deviation of the *differences*. This is much harder to estimate than the standard deviation of the individual observations. A pilot study is usually indicated.

    The N in the nomogram represents the number of pairs of observations required in the experiment. If each pair represents two matched patients, the number of patients required is $2N$.

- *Comparing two proportions*. The *chi-square test* or, equivalently, a standardized *Normal deviate* is used to test the null hypothesis that the proportion of individuals possessing a certain attribute is the same in two groups. The response variable in this instance is a binary categorical variable. The standardized difference is

$$\frac{p_1 - p_2}{\sqrt{\{\bar{p}(1-\bar{p})\}}}$$

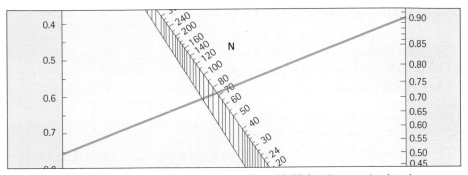

Fig. 4 The line produced by connecting the value of 0.75 for the standardized difference to the power value of 0.90 cuts the axis for a significance level of 0.05 at about $N = 70$ (a magnified section of Fig. I is shown)

where:

$p_1 - p_2$ is the difference between the proportions of individuals with the attribute, that, if it really existed, would be considered clinically important.

$\bar{p}$ is the mean of p_1 and p_2.

The $N = 2n$ in the nomogram represents the total number of individuals required in the sample, with n in each group.

As an example, suppose it is of interest to establish the optimal sample size for a proposed study which will compare, in a given district, the dental fluorosis rates in children aged between 5 and 18 who have been either lifelong consumers of moderate- to high-fluoride surface water (0·50 mg F/L) or low-fluoride surface water (approximately 0·10 mg F/L). It is believed that the dental fluorosis rate in the low fluoride group is about 15%. A difference between the two groups in fluorosis rates of about 35% would be regarded as clinically important. In this case, $\bar{p} = 32·5\%$ and the standardized difference is $(50 - 15)/\sqrt{(32·5 \times 67·5)} = 0·75$. Note that percentages have been used instead of proportions in this example, so the 'one' in the denominator of the standardized difference is replaced by '100'. Thus, by using the nomogram, it can be seen that in order to have a power of 90% of detecting a difference of 35% in fluorosis rates at the 5% level of significance about 70 children would be required (Fig. 4), with approximately 35 in each of the fluoride groups.

Sequential analysis

The methods discussed so far for determining the optimal sample size in an experiment relate to **fixed sample size** designs. It is assumed that the total sample size is a finite number which is fixed before the experiment is started. It is chosen in accordance with relevant power considerations, but also with reference to the expected patient accrual rate and the proposed time of investigation and costs.

As an alternative approach, the patients can be entered *one at a time* into the clinical trial, and their responses, as they occur, can be used to test the hypothesis of interest. Either the trial is stopped in favour of one of the treatments when a significant treatment effect is observed; or it is stopped when it is considered that that no treatment difference is likely to arise. In both cases, the decision to stop is made with reference to a chart which is constructed by considering the significance level, the power and the size of the effect, all of which are specified at the outset. Clearly, in such a **sequential** trial (Armitage, 1975),[4] there is no need to estimate the patient numbers at the design stage, because the sample size depends on the results.

The advantage of a sequential trial is that it requires less patients than its fixed sample size counterpart if there is a large treatment effect. However, sequential trials are rarely performed, mostly because they are restricted to conditions in which there is only one response and when the time required to observe the response to treatment is not prolonged. Furthermore, it can be difficult to estimate the effect of interest and provide confidence intervals in a sequential study.

Interim analyses

Sometimes clinical trials are designed so that the investigators can check the results at one or more *predefined* intermediate stages; these trials are often called **group sequential trials.** Apart from ensuring that the trial is running smoothly as regards compliance and that there is no concern about side-effects, the investigators may wish to perform significance tests to evaluate treatment effects at these times. Then, if one treatment is found to be superior, the trial can be stopped early and all the patients will go on to receive the most effective treatment.

Clearly, there are ethical advantages to this approach. However, be warned that such a proposal is not as straightforward as it might at first appear, and it is open to criticism if the statistical methods are not handled appropriately.

The problem with performing significance tests at intermediate stages is that the significance level at the end of the trial is larger than it would be if there were no repeated tests. In other words, there will be a greater chance of concluding that there is a significant difference between treatments when in reality there is no difference between them. Hence it is necessary to adjust the significance levels used for the intermediate or interim analyses to ensure that the final significance level is as expected, typically 0·05 or, perhaps, 0·01. Pocock (1983)[5] provides a table which shows, under certain conditions, which significance level to use at each intermediate stage (this is called the *nominal significance level*) if the significance level at the final stage (this is called the *overall significance level*) is 0·05 or 0·01. For example, if there were to be five repeated significance tests, the nominal level for each should be 0·016 (ie each repeated test is significant if $P < 0·016$) in order to have the overall significance level at 0·05.

1   *nQueryAdvisor Version 5.0* Statistical Solutions Ltd.
2   Machin D, Campbell M J, Fayers P M, Pinol A P Y. *Sample Size Tables for Clinical Studies.* 2nd edn. Oxford: Blackwell Science, 1997.
3   Altman D G. How large a sample? *Statistics in Practice* (eds Gore S.M. and Altman D.G.) British Medical Association, London, 1982
4   Armitage P. *Sequential Medical Trials.* 2nd edn. Oxford: Blackwell Scientific Publications, 1975.
5   Pocock S J. *Clinical Trials: a Practical Approach.* Wiley, Chichester, 1983.

Diagnostic tests for oral conditions

A diagnostic test is a simple test, sometimes based on a clinical measurement, which is used when the gold-standard test providing a definitive diagnosis of a given condition is too expensive, invasive or time-consuming to perform. The diagnostic test can be used to diagnose a dental condition in an individual patient or as a screening device in a population of apparently healthy individuals.

When clinicians want to make a **diagnosis** for a particular patient, they are often faced with a number of possibilities. A diagnostic test, usually performed in conjunction with a clinical examination, may be used to exclude some diagnoses or categorise the patient as either having or not having a specific disease. Such a diagnosis is rarely definitive but it is possible for the clinician to use the test result to decide whether a disease is unlikely or probable in a particular patient. Diagnostic tests can also be used for **screening**, the objective of which is to determine whether members of an apparently healthy target population are likely to have the disease or condition under investigation. Often the screening test will be a first step in selecting people likely to have the condition, and this may be confirmed later using more refined procedures. The reasoning is that if such conditions can be easily detected in the early, pre-symptomatic stages, then subsequent treatment, cure, or prevention may be easier, less costly, and may have a better chance of succeeding.

A diagnostic test may suggest that a disease (eg oral cancer) is present on the basis of a *categorical outcome* (eg whether or not a red patch, white patch or ulcer of greater than 2 week's duration can be detected (Downer *et al.*, 1995)).[1] Sometimes the diagnostic test is based on a *continuous* measurement and the patient classified as having some disease if the level of the measurement exceeds (or is less than) a particular value, the **cut-off** value. For example, there is a suggestion (Streckfus *et al.*, 2001) that it might be possible to use the concentrations of the salivary protein c-*erb*B-2 as a marker for the initial detection and follow-up screening for the recurrence of breast cancer in men and women.[2] The cut-off is usually the upper (or the lower) limit of the reference range for that measurement. The reference range is the range of values which includes a large proportion (usually 95%) of the healthy (disease-free) individuals in the population. If the cut-off is set too low (in the instance in which high levels of the measurement indicate disease) then some people will be classified as having the disease when, in reality, they are disease-free. This can be costly in terms of money, time and the unnecessary psychological stress induced. If, however, the cut-off is set too high then patients with the disease will be missed, and this may have dire consequences for the individual, or in the case of an infectious disease, others in the population. An approach to choosing the optimal cut-off is explained in greater depth later in the last section of this chapter.

The philosophy of screening

On the face of it, the concept of screening seems entirely laudable providing, of course, that suitable diagnostic tests exist. However, there are several points which have to be carefully considered. There may be serious ethical considerations. When an individual patient seeks help from a doctor or dentist, the implication is that any advice or treatment is being provided at the request of the patient. In a screening exercise, however, the initiative may not come from the patient, but from the doctor or dentist proposing the screening. In other words, it is not the patient making the first move by saying to the dentist *'I think I have something wrong with me — please do what you can to help me'* but rather the dentist making the first move by saying to the patient *'Although you have no symptoms of the disease now, the result of this test could indicate that you may have a problem which could be treated'.*

It follows that if further investigation and treatment are being offered to patients following the positive result of a screening test, then the practitioner must be sure that:

- Adequate facilities for such investigation or treatment are available.
- There is an agreed policy on the stage in the disease process at which active treatment is needed.
- The proposed treatment will actually benefit the patient.
- Adequate funds are available to cover the costs involved.

- The subjects tested fully understand the implications of the result of a positive test. So, for example, if a child scored positive in a school screening for dental caries it would be wrong to say 'This examination has shown that you need dental treatment', but more correct to say 'This examination has indicated that you could probably benefit from a more detailed examination by your own, or the school, dentist, if you have not had such an examination recently.'

Furthermore, before a mass screening procedure is implemented, the organisers need to satisfy themselves that:

- The disease or condition constitutes an important public health problem. This means either a condition with a high prevalence in the population, such as dental caries, or a condition which although not commanding a high prevalence is so serious as to be life-threatening or disabling, such as oral cancer.

- The cost of the screening programme for a relatively minor condition is not going to divert resources needed for the routine treatment of more serious conditions.

- The condition under investigation lends itself to screening, in that there is a recognisable latent or early symptomatic stage in the disease process. Dental caries, periodontal disease and oral cancer all clearly fulfil this criterion.

- A satisfactory and viable screening test exists. This should be:
  i) *Cheap*: that is, with a low per-capita cost, for obvious reasons.
  ii) *Fast*: since lengthy tests mean not only that subjects will be reluctant to participate, but also that operative costs per capita will be greatly increased and the disease may progress.
  iii) *Acceptable*: in other words non-invasive, painless and not subjecting the subjects in any way to embarrassment or humiliation.
  iv) *Reliable*: in that different operators will always obtain similar results on the same subjects.

Sensitivity and specificity of a test

Diagnostic tests used for both diagnosis and screening need to have a high degree of **validity**, and it is here that statistical analysis comes in. Validity in this context means the ability of the test to fulfil the required objectives; to indicate the presence of the disease or condition (ie to give a **positive** test result) for those with it, and to give a **negative** test result for those who are free of it.

An ideal test for a given condition would, of course, be positive for every person in whom the condition was present, and negative for those in whom it was absent. Sadly, this ideal is rarely, if ever, achieved. If it were perfect, the test would not be a test in this sense, but the gold standard diagnosis. Some tests will accurately identify all the positive cases, but only at the expense of returning a **false positive** result on some individuals who are free of the condition. Other tests may successfully identify all those who are free of the condition, but may also miss some of those who actually have it, returning a **false negative** result on some individuals with the disease. And others may be less than 100% successful in both directions.

In order to provide a measure of the relative validity of diagnostic and screening tests, the terms sensitivity and specificity have come into use.

Sensitivity is the probability (usually expressed as a percentage) that a subject with the disease will have a positive test result. With a perfect test, all those with the disease will have a positive test result and the sensitivity will then be 100%. A test with low sensitivity will fail to indicate disease in many of those that have it. The rate at which this occurs is called the *false negative rate*; sensitivity is equal to one hundred minus the false negative rate.

Specificity is the probability (usually expressed as a percentage) that a subject who is free of the disease will have a negative test result. Once again, with a perfect test all those free of the disease will have a negative test result and the specificity of that test will be 100%. A test with low specificity will falsely indicate the presence of disease in many of those that are free of it. The rate at which this occurs is called the *false positive rate*; specificity is equal to one hundred minus the false positive rate.

In algebraic terms:

$$\text{Sensitivity} = Pr(\text{T+}|\text{D+})$$
$$\text{Specificity} = Pr(\text{T-}|\text{D-})$$

where $Pr(A|B)$ is the probability of A given that B is true and is called a conditional probability. $Pr(\text{T+}|\text{D+})$ therefore indicates the probability that the test (T) is positive, given that the disease (D) is positive (ie present).

Table I Table of frequencies showing the results of a screening test		
	D+	D–
T+	17	29
T–	99	396
Total	116	425

Example

Even though preventative programmes against dental disease are extremely effective, there are still individuals who develop large numbers of caries lesions. A screening programme for the early detection of these potentially high-risk individuals is useful in that special preventative programmes can be instituted for them which will result in a low cost-effectiveness ratio. Several micro-organisms have high cariogenic potential and have served as a basis for identifying individuals susceptible to caries. In particular, the level of lactobacilli has been shown to have a positive association with the incidence of dental caries. A 17-month long longitudinal study (Kingman et al., 1988)[3] of 541 US adolescents initially aged 10–15 years was conducted with a view to establishing a screening test for high risk individuals, taking a bacterial level of lactobacilli $>10^5$ as a positive test result. A saliva sample was taken from every subject at baseline and the number of lactobacilli recorded. These measurements were related to the caries increment after 17 months, where at least three new lesions in the period was recorded as a positive disease result. Of the 541 children screened, 116 actually were disease positive after 17 months and 425 were disease negative. It is possible to display these results in a 2 × 2 contingency table of frequencies (Table 1):

This table indicates that the test successfully identifies 17 of the 116 subjects with the disease as positive, but records the remaining 99 falsely as negative. Similarly, it successfully identifies 396 of the 425 disease-free children, but gives a false positive result for the remaining 29.

From this table it is possible to calculate:

Sensitivity = 17/116 = 0·147 (ie 14·7% or approximately 15%)
Specificity = 396/425 = 0·932 (ie 93·2% or approximately 93%)

Thus there is a 15% chance that, using this test, a child with disease will screen positive, and a 93% chance that a child who is disease-free will screen negative.

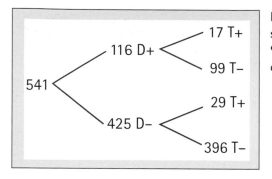

Fig. I Tree diagram for a test with sensitivity= 14·7%, specificity = 93·2% and estimated prevalence of disease = 21·4%

Positive and negative predictive values

At this stage it is necessary to refer to a popular misconception, which is to assume that just because a test has a sensitivity of 15%, it follows that a child who screens positive has a 15% chance of having the disease. To show that this is not the case, consider a tree diagram (Fig. 1) which displays the same results as those in Table 1. This diagram clearly shows that although 46 children test positive, only 17 of them have the disease. Thus if a child screens positive, the probability that he/she will have the disease is 17/(17 + 29) = 0·370 or 37%, which is substantially greater than the sensitivity of 15%.

It is now possible to introduce two new terms, both of which assess the usefulness of the test in practice:

The **positive predictive value (PPV)** which is the probability (usually expressed as a percentage) that an individual who has a positive test result actually has the disease. In algebraic terms, PPV = $Pr(D+|T+)$ which is 37·0% in the caries example.

The **negative predictive value (NPV)** which is the probability (usually expressed as a percentage) that someone who has a negative test result does not have the disease. In algebraic terms, NPV = $Pr(D-|T-)$ which is 80·0% in the caries example.

Further investigation along these lines shows that the positive predictive value and the negative predictive value of a test depend both on the sensitivity and specificity of the test and also on the **prevalence** of the disease in the population. The prevalence of a disease is the proportion of individuals in the population who have the disease, which, in the context of a screening test, is taken as the *pre-test* probability or *a priori* probability that an individual has the disease. For a given test, the positive predictive value will be greater when

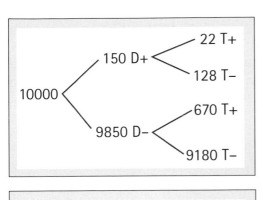

Fig. 2 (a) Tree diagram for a test with sensitivity = 14.7%, specificity = 93.2% and estimated prevalence = 1.5%

Fig. 2 (b) Tree diagram for a test with sensitivity = 14.7%, specificity = 45.2% and estimated prevalence = 21.4%

the prevalence is high than when the disease prevalence is low. The reverse is true for the negative predictive value. Note that the sensitivity and specificity of a test are not affected by the prevalence of the condition. The prevalence is estimated in the sample by p which is D+ divided by the total number of individuals in the sample; so $p = 116/541 = 0 \cdot 214$ (ie approximately 21%).

The calculations of the PPV and NPV shown in this paper require knowledge of the diagnostic test result as well as the true diagnosis in every member of a group of individuals. A later chapter, Bayesian Statistics, describes an alternative method clinicians can use in order to determine the PPV of a test if they only have knowledge of the pre-test probability of the disease and the test result for a given patient. In these circumstances, the PPV is usually called the *post-test* or *posterior* probability of the disease.

As an illustration of the relationship between the positive predictive value of a test and the prevalence of a disease, consider a sample of 10,000 children from a different population; the disease prevalence (ie a caries incidence of at least 3 new DMFS) in this population is only 1·5%. If the sensitivity and specificity of the test remain at 14·7% and 93·2% respectively, a quick calculation will show (Fig. 2a) that of the 150 children with the disease, 22 will screen positive and 128 will screen negative; of those 9,850 without the disease, 670 will screen positive and 9,180 will screen negative. Thus if a child screens positive, there would be a 22/692 = 0·032 or 3·2% chance that he/she has the disease, ie the PPV = (22)/(22 + 670) = 0·032. Hence, for this lactobacilli test, the PPV is reduced from 37% when the prevalence is 21% to approximately 3% when the prevalence is only 1·5%. The reverse is true for the NPV which increases from 80% to approximately 99% in these circumstances.

This result indicates the important difference between a diagnostic test when it is used for screening and diagnosis. Even if precisely the same test is used, when it is applied to screen a population which is apparently healthy (with respect to the disease or condition being studied), the *a priori* or pre-test probability of having the disease (ie the prevalence) is low. In this case, the positive predictive value or post-test probability is also likely to be low. On the other hand, if a patient complains to his doctor or dentist about a series of symptoms, and a case history leads the doctor or dentist to formulate a hypothesis that the patient has a certain disease, the probability that the hypothesis is correct should be relatively high before the test is performed, and a positive test result acts as a confirmation of the diagnosis. If, for example, with all the information given by the patient, the doctor or dentist thinks (with probability, say 0·75) that the patient has disease X, the predictive value of a positive test may be close to 100%. A good clinician formulates a hypothesis (and maybe an alternative) and requests one or two diagnostic tests. Note that a less skilled clinician might have no clear idea of the cause of the patient's problem, and may request a long battery of tests, not realising that, if a large number of tests are performed, there is a high probability that something will turn up positive purely by chance.

In order to investigate the relationship between the positive predictive value and specificity, consider a different test (relating to the level of *mutans streptococci*, say) in the first sample of children for whom the estimated disease prevalence is 21·4%; suppose that the sensitivity of this test is also 14·7% but its specificity is only 45·2% (Fig. 2b) rather than the 93·2% obtained for the lactobacilli test. Here (17 + 233) children test positive of whom only 17 have the disease. So if a child screens positive, the chance of him/her having the disease (ie his/her positive predictive value) is only 17/(17 + 233) = 0·068. Thus (rounding the percentages), if the prevalence (21%) and the sensitivity (15%)

Table 2 Table of frequencies with frequencies expressed in general terms

	D+	D–	Total
T+	a (true positive)	b (false positive)	a+b
T–	c (false negative)	d (true negative)	c+d
Total	a+c	b+d	n

remain unaltered, a test with a specificity of 45% instead of 93% lowers the PPV from 37% to 7%.

Calculations of the measures of the test effectiveness

The calculations for these statistics, which are estimates of the true population values, may now be summarised using the notation of Table 2, a generalised 2 × 2 table of frequencies:

Sensitivity = $Pr(\text{T+}|\text{D+}) = a/(a + c)$
Specificity = $Pr(\text{T–}|\text{D–}) = d/(b + d)$
Positive Predictive Value = $Pr(\text{D+}|\text{T+}) = a/(a + b)$
Negative Predictive Value = $Pr(\text{D–}|\text{T–}) = d/(c + d)$
Prevalence, $p = (a + c)/n$ (This is the pre-test or *a priori* probability of having the condition)

Finally, it may be of interest to obtain an estimate of the prevalence of the condition if the sensitivity and specificity of the test are known (and expressed as probabilities), and $Pr(\text{T+})$ is the proportion of individuals in the sample testing positive. Then,

$$p = \frac{\text{Specificity} + Pr(\text{T+}) - 1}{\text{Sensitivity} + \text{Specificity} - 1}$$

that is, if sensitivity = specificity = 0.9, and 12% of the sample test positive, then the estimated prevalence is:

$$p = \frac{0.9 + 0.12 - 1}{0.9 + 0.9 - 1} = 0.025 \text{ (ie 2·5%)}$$

It is a näive mistake to confuse the proportion who have a positive test result with the prevalence of the disease. As shown above, if 12% of the tests are positive, this does not mean that 12% of the individuals have the disease!

Note that the sensitivity, specificity and positive and negative predictive values of a test are generally evaluated using sample data and are only estimates of their true values in the population. It is possible, using the statistical theory of the binomial distribution, to calculate the standard errors of the estimates, and use the latter to determine confidence intervals for the population values.

Choosing a test

Although the aim should be to devise a test which has both a high sensitivity and a high specificity, it must be recognised that often one has to be sacrificed in order to accommodate the other since they are inversely related, sensitivity increasing as the specificity decreases and *vice versa*. Hence it is necessary in any given situation to establish what is required from the test and the consequences of false positive and false negative results. For example, if the test is to be used to screen for a fatal non-infectious disease, then it is important to be able to reassure individuals that they do not have the disease and avoid the risk of false positives; here, specificity and the NPV are of prime importance. If, on the other hand, the disease is treatable but infectious, it will be important for the screening test to have high sensitivity, ensuring that the false negative rate is low and not many true cases of the disease are missed. A confirmatory test with high specificity, and therefore a low false positive rate, can then be used on those individuals who were positive on the initial screen. If the test is based on a continuous measurement so that a test result is positive if an individual's value exceeds (say) a particular cut-off value for the measurement, then it is possible to alter the sensitivity and specificity of the test by changing the cut-off. If this cut-off is raised, fewer individuals with the disease will be classified as positive, the sensitivity will decrease and there will be more false negatives. At the same time, more individuals will appear to be disease-free so that the specificity will increase and there will be less false positives. If the cut-off for this measurement is lowered, the reverse is true and the sensitivity will increase and the specificity will decrease.

As an illustration of these concepts, consider the lactobacilli example for the detection of potentially high risk caries children. When a bacterial level of $> 10^5$ was chosen as the cut-off, the sensitivity and specificity of the test were approximately 15% and 93%, respectively. However, when a level $> 10^6$ was chosen as the cut-off, fewer high risk children were identified and the sensitivity and specificity of the test were 2% and nearly 100%, respectively. On the other

52

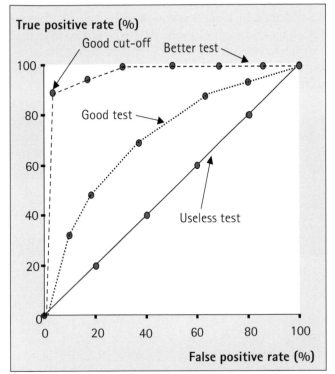

hand, when a level $> 10^2$ was chosen as the cut-off, the sensitivity and specificity of the test were 79% and 50%, respectively.

In order to decide on an optimal cut-off for a given test, it is possible to draw its **receiver operating characteristic** (ROC) curve. If rates are expressed as percentages, this is a plot (Fig. 3) of the sensitivity (ie the true positive rate equal to 100 minus the false negative rate) on the vertical axis against 100 minus the specificity (ie the false positive rate) on the horizontal axis for various cut-off values for the measurement. If the true and false positive rates are equal for all cut-off values for a test, the resulting curve is a diagonal straight line from the bottom left-hand corner to the top-right hand corner. The ROC curve should never pass below the diagonal, as this would imply that the false positive rate is greater than the true positive rate. Choosing a cut-off from the ROC depends on the specific requirements of the test and the implications of false negative and false positive results The perfect cut-off for any test is one which produces no false positives and no false negatives and so is the point at the top left hand corner of the ROC diagram. If a very good test can be regarded as that with a high true positive rate and consequently very few false negatives, its curve would rise steeply from the bottom left-hand corner, almost reaching the top-left-hand corner, before flattening out. It is possible to use the ROC curve to choose the optimal cut-off value for a particular test by specifying the required sensitivity and specificity of the test, a non-statistical decision based on the clinical implications of a false negative and false positive result. In addition, two or more tests may be compared by evaluating the area under each of the ROC curves; generally, the test with the greater area is the 'better' test overall.

1   Downer M C, Evans A W, Hughes Hallet C M, Jullien J A, Speight P M, Zakrzewska J M. Evaluation of screening for oral cancer and precancer in a company headquarters. *Community Dent Oral Epidemiol* 1995; 2 3: 84-88.
2   Streckfus C, Bigler L, Dellinger T, Dai X, Cox W J, McArthur A, Kingman A, Thigpen J T. Reliability assessment of soluble c-erbB-2 concentrations in the saliva of healthy women and men. *Oral Med* 2001; 9 1: 174-179.
3   Kingman A, Little W, Gomez I, Heifetz S B, Driscoll W S, Sheats R, Supan P. Salivary levels of Streptococcus mutans and lactobacilli and dental caries experiences in a US adolescent population. *Community Dent Oral Epidemiol* 1988; 1 6: 98-103.

Multiple linear regression

6

In order to introduce the concepts underlying multiple linear regression, it is necessary to be familiar with and understand the basic theory of simple linear regression on which it is based.

Reviewing simple linear regression

Simple linear regression analysis is concerned with describing the linear relationship between a dependent (outcome) variable, y, and single explanatory (independent or predictor) variable, x. Full details may be obtained from texts such as Bulman and Osborn (1989),[1] Chatterjee and Price (1999)[2] and Petrie and Sabin (2000).[3]

Suppose that each individual in a sample of size n has a pair of values, one for x and one for y; it is assumed that y depends on x, rather than the other way round. It is helpful to start by plotting the data in a **scatter diagram** (Fig. 1a), conventionally putting x on the horizontal axis and y on the vertical axis. The resulting scatter of the points will indicate whether or not a linear relationship is sensible, and may pinpoint outliers which would distort the analysis. If appropriate, this linear relationship can be described by an equation defining the line (Fig. 1b), the regression of y on x, which is given by:

$$Y = \alpha + \beta x$$

This is estimated in the sample by:

$$Y = a + bx$$

where:

Y is the predicted value of the dependent variable, y, for a particular value of the explanatory variable, x

a is the intercept of the estimated line (the value of Y when $x = 0$), estimating the true value, α, in the population

b is the slope, gradient or regression coefficient of the estimated line (the average change in y for a unit change in x), estimating the true value, β, in the population.

The parameters which define the line, namely the **intercept** (estimated by a, and often not of inherent interest) and the **slope** (estimated by b) need to be examined. In particular, **standard errors** can be estimated, **confidence intervals** can be determined for them, and, if required, the confidence intervals for the points and/or the line can be drawn. Interest is usually focused on the **slope** of the line which determines the extent to which y varies as x is increased. If the slope is zero, then changing x has no effect on y, and there is no linear relationship between the two variables. A t-test can be used to test the null hypothesis that the true slope is zero, the test statistic being:

$$t = \frac{b}{SE(b)}$$

which approximately follows the t-distribution on $n-2$ degrees of freedom. If a relationship exists (ie there is a significant slope), the line can be used to **predict** the value of the dependent variable from a value of the explanatory variable by substituting the latter value into the estimated equation. It must be remembered that the estimated line is only valid in the range of values for which there are observations on x and y.

The correlation coefficient is a measure of linear association between two variables. Its true value in the population, ρ, is estimated in the sample by r. The correlation coefficient takes a value between and including minus one and plus one, its sign denoting the direction of the slope of the line. It is possible to perform a significance test (Fig. 1a) on the null hypothesis that $\rho = 0$, the situation in which there is no linear association between the variables. Because of the mathematical relationship between the correlation coefficient and the slope of the regression line, if the slope is significantly different from zero, then the correlation coefficient will be too. However, this is not to say that the line is a good 'fit' to the data points as there may be considerable scatter about the line even if the correlation coefficient is significantly different from zero. **Goodness-of-fit** can be investigated by calculating r^2, the square of the estimated correlation coefficient. It describes

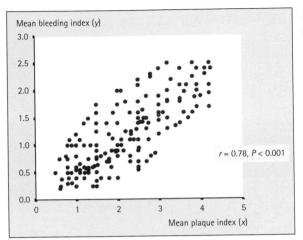

Fig. 1a Scatter diagram showing the relationship between the mean bleeding index per child and the mean plaque index per child in a sample of 170 12-year-old schoolchildren (derived from data kindly provided by Dr Gareth Griffiths of the Eastman Dental Institute for Oral Health Care Sciences, University College London)

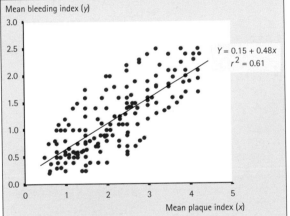

Fig. 1b Estimated linear regression line of the mean bleeding index against the mean plaque index using the data of Fig. 1a. Intercept, $a = 0.15$; slope, $b = 0.48$ (95% CI $= 0.42$ to 0.54, $P < 0.001$), indicating that the mean bleeding index increases on average by 0.48 as the mean plaque index increases by one

the proportion of the variability of y that can be attributed to or be explained by the linear relationship between x and y; it is usually multiplied by 100 and expressed as a percentage. A subjective evaluation leads to a decision as to whether or not the line is a good fit. For example, a value of 61% (Fig. 1b) indicates that a substantial percentage of the variability of y is explained by the regression of y on x — only 39% is unexplained by the relationship — and such a line would be regarded as a reasonably good fit. On the other hand, if $r^2 = 0.25$ then 75% of the variability of y is unexplained by the relationship, and the line is a poor fit.

The multiple linear regression equation

Multiple linear regression (usually simply called multiple regression) may be regarded as an extension to simple linear regression when more than one explanatory variable is included in the regression model. For each individual, there is information on his or her values for the outcome variable, y, and each of k, say, explanatory variables, $x_1, x_2, ..., x_k$. Usually, focus is centred on determining whether a particular explanatory variable, x_i, has a significant effect on y after adjusting for the effects of the other explanatory variables. Furthermore, it is possible to assess the joint effect of these k explanatory variables on y, by formulating an appropriate model which can then be used to predict values of y for a particular combination of explanatory variables.

The multiple linear regression equation in the population is described by the relationship:

$$Y = \alpha + \beta_1 x_1 + \beta_2 x_2 + ... + \beta_k x_k$$

This is estimated in the sample by:

$$Y = a + b_1 x_1 + b_2 x_2 + ... + b_k x_k$$

where:

Y is the predicted value of the dependent variable, y, for a particular set of values of explanatory variables, $x_1, x_2, ..., x_k$.

a is a constant term (the 'intercept', the value of Y when all the x's are zero), estimating the true value, α, in the population

b_i is the estimated partial regression coefficient (the average change in y for a unit change in x_i, adjusting for all the other x's), estimating the true value, β_i, in the population. It is usually simply called the regression coefficient. It will be different from the regression coefficient obtained from the simple linear regression of y on x_i alone if the explanatory variables are interrelated. The multiple regression equation adjusts for the effects of the explanatory variables, and this will only be necessary if they are correlated. Note that although the explanatory variables are often called 'independent' variables, this terminology gives a false impression, as the explanatory variables are rarely independent of each other.

In this computer age, multiple regression is rarely performed by hand, and so this chapter does not include formulae for the regression coefficients and their standard errors. If computer output from a particular statistical package omits confidence intervals for the coefficients, the 95% confidence interval for β_i can be calculated as $b_i \pm t_{0.05}\, \text{SE}(b_i)$, where $t_{0.05}$ is the percentage point of the t-distribution which corresponds to a two-tailed probability of 0.05, and $\text{SE}(b_i)$ is the estimated standard error of b_i.

Computer output in a multiple regression analysis

Being able to use the appropriate computer software for a multiple regression analysis is usually relatively easy, as long as it is possible to distinguish between the dependent and explanatory variables, and the terminology is familiar. Knowing how to interpret the output may pose more of a problem; different statistical packages produce varying output, some more elaborate than others, and it is essential that one is able to select those results which are useful and can interpret them.

Goodness-of-fit

In *simple linear regression*, the square of the correlation coefficient, r^2, can be used to measure the 'goodness-of-fit' of the model. r^2 represents the proportion of the variability of y that can be explained by its linear relationship with x, a large value suggesting that the model is a good fit. The approach used in *multiple linear regression* is similar to that in simple linear regression. A quantity, R^2, sometimes called the coefficient of determination, describes the proportion of the total variability of y which is explained by the linear relationship of y on all the x's, and gives an indication of the goodness-of-fit of a model. However, it is inappropriate to compare the values of R^2 from multiple regression equations which have differing numbers of explanatory variables, as the value of R^2 will be greater for those models which contain a larger number of explanatory variables. So, instead, an **adjusted** R^2 value is used in these circumstances. Assessing the goodness-of-fit of a model is more important when the aim is to use the regression model for prediction than when it is used to assess the effect of each of the explanatory variables on the outcome variable.

Table I Analysis of variance table for the regression analysis of OHQoL					
Source of variation	Sum of squares	Degrees of freedom	Mean square	F	P-value
Regression	3618.480	9	402.053	5.678	<0.001
Residual	10693.073	151	70.815		
Total	14311.553	160			

The analysis of variance table

A comprehensive computer output from a multiple regression analysis will include an analysis of variance (ANOVA) table (Table 1). This is used to assess whether at least one of the explanatory variables has a significant linear relationship with the dependent variable. The null hypothesis is that *all* the partial regression coefficients in the model are zero. The ANOVA table partitions the total variance of the dependent variable, y, into two components; that which is due to the relationship of y with all the x's, and that which is left over afterwards, termed the residual variance. These two variances are compared in the table by calculating their ratio which follows the F-distribution so that a P-value can be determined. If the P-value is small (say, less than 0·05), it is unlikely that the null hypothesis is true.

Assessing the effect of each explanatory variable on outcome

If the result of the F-test from the analysis of variance table is significant (ie typically if $P < 0·05$), indicating that at least one of the explanatory variables is independently associated with the outcome variable, it is necessary to establish which of the variables is a useful predictor of outcome. Each of the regression coefficients in the model can be tested (the null hypothesis is that the true coefficient is zero in the population) using a test statistic which follows the t-distribution with $n - k - 1$ degrees of freedom, where n is the sample size and k is the number of explanatory variables in the model. This test statistic is similar to that used in simple linear regression, ie it is the ratio of the estimated coefficient to its standard error. Computer output contains a table (Table 2) which usually shows the constant term and estimated partial regression coefficients (a and the b's) with their standard errors (with, perhaps, confidence intervals for the true partial regression coefficients), the test statistic for each coefficient, and the resulting P-value. From this information, the multiple regression equation can be formulated, and a decision made as to which of the explanatory variables are significantly independently associated with outcome. A particular partial regression coefficient, b_1 say, represents the average change in y for a unit change in x_1, after adjusting for the other explanatory variables in the equation. If the equation is required for prediction, then the analysis can be re-run using only those variables which are significant, and a new multiple regression equation created; this will probably have partial regression coefficients which differ slightly from those of the original larger model.

Table 2 Results of multiple regression analysis with OHQoL as the dependent variable

Model	Estimated coefficient				95% confidence interval for regression coefficient	
	b	Std. Error	Test statistic	P-value	Lower bound	Upper bound
(Constant)	52·583	4·734	11·108	< 0·001	43·230	61·936
Gender (0 = F, 1 = M)	−2·832	1·387	−2·041	0·043	−5·574	−0·091
Age*	2·965	2·198	1·349	0·179	−1·378	7·307
Social class†	−3·282	1·542	−2·128	0·035	−6·329	−0·234
Toothache (0 = N, 1 = Y)	−5·600	1·543	−3·629	< 0·001	−8·648	−2·551
Broken teeth (0 = N, 1 = Y)	−2·526	1·554	−1·625	0·106	−5·596	0·544
Broken/ill fitting denture¥	−3·079	1·792	−1·719	0·088	−6·619	0·461
Sore or bleeding gums in last year∫	−1·791	1·540	−1·163	0·247	−4·834	1·252
Loose teeth (0 = N, 1 = Y)	−4·020	2·262	−1·777	0·078	−8·489	0·449
Tooth health#	0·079	0·038	2·106	0·037	0·005	0·153

*(0 = under 55yrs, 1 = 55yrs or more)
†(1 = 1,11,111NM, 2 = 111M, 1V, V)
¥(0 = N, 1 = Y) ∫(0 = N, 1 = Y)
#Explained in the text

Automatic model selection procedures

It is important, when choosing which explanatory variables to include in a model, not to over-fit the model by including too many of them. Whilst explaining the data very well, an over-fitted or, in particular, a saturated model (ie one in which there are as many explanatory variables as individuals in the sample) is usually of little use for predicting future outcomes. It is generally accepted that a sensible model should include no more than $n/10$ explanatory variables, where n is the number of individuals in the sample. Put another way, there should be at least ten times as many individuals in the sample as variables in the model.

When there are only a limited number of variables that are of interest, they are usually all included in the model. The difficulty arises when there are a relatively large number of potential explanatory variables, all of which are scientifically reasonable, and it seems sensible to include only some of them in the model. The most usual approach is to establish which explanatory variables are significantly (perhaps at the 10% or even 20% level rather than the more usual 5% level) related to the outcome variable when each is investigated separately, ignoring the other explanatory variables in the study. Then only these 'significant' variables are included in the model. So, if the explanatory variable is binary, this might involve performing a two-sample t-test to determine whether the mean value of the outcome variable is different in the two categories of the explanatory variable. If the explanatory variable is continuous, then a significant slope in a simple linear regression analysis would suggest that this variable should be included in the multiple regression model.

If the purpose of the multiple regression analysis is to gain some understanding of the relationship between the outcome and explanatory variables and an insight into the independent effects of each of the latter on the former, then entering all relevant variables into the model is the way to proceed. However, sometimes the purpose of the analysis is to obtain the most appropriate model which can be used for predicting the outcome variable. One approach in this situation is to put all the relevant explanatory variables into the model, observe which are significant, and obtain a final condensed multiple regression model by re-running the analysis using only these significant variables. The alternative approach is to use an **automatic selection procedure**, offered by most statistical packages, to select the optimal combination of explanatory variables in a prescribed manner. In particular, one of the following procedures can be chosen:

- **All subsets selection** — every combination of explanatory variables is investigated and that which provides the best fit, as described by the value of some criterion such as the adjusted R^2, is selected.

- **Forwards (step-up) selection** — the first step is to create a simple model with one explanatory variable which gives the best R^2 when compared to all other models with only one variable. In the next step, a second variable is added to the existing model if it is better than any other variable at explaining the remaining variability and produces a model which is significantly better (according to some criterion) than that in the previous step. This process is repeated progressively until the addition of a further variable does not significantly improve the model.

- **Backwards (step-down) selection** — the first step is to create the full model which includes all the variables. The next step is to remove the least significant variable from the model, and retain this reduced model if it is not significantly worse (according to some criterion) than the model in the previous step. This process is repeated progressively, stopping when the removal of a variable is significantly detrimental.

- **Stepwise selection** — this is a combination of forwards and backwards selection. Essentially it is forwards selection, but it allows variables which have been included in the model to be removed, by checking that all of the included variables are still required.

It is important to note that these automatic selection procedures may lead to different models, particularly if the explanatory variables are highly correlated, ie when there is collinearity. In these circumstances, deciding on the model can be problematic, and this may be compounded by the fact that the resulting models, although mathematically legitimate, may not be sensible. It is crucial, therefore, to apply common sense and be able to justify the model in a biological and/or clinical context when selecting the most appropriate model.

Including categorical variables in the model

1. Categorical explanatory variables
It is possible to include categorical explanatory variables in a multiple regression model. If the explanatory variable is **binary** or **dichotomous**, then a numerical code is chosen for the two responses, typically 0 and 1. So for example, if gender

is one of the explanatory variables, then females might be coded as 0 and males as 1. This **dummy** variable is entered into the model in the usual way as if it were a numerical variable. The estimated partial regression coefficient for the dummy variable is interpreted as the average change in y for a unit change in the dummy variable, after adjusting for the other explanatory variables in the model. Thus in the example, it is difference in the estimated mean values of y in males and females, a positive difference indicating that the mean is greater for males than females.

If the two categories of the binary explanatory variable represent different treatments, then including this variable in the multiple regression equation is a particular approach to what is termed the **analysis of covariance**. Using a multiple regression analysis, the effect of treatment can be assessed on the outcome variable, after adjusting for the other explanatory variables in the model.

When the explanatory variable is qualitative and it has **more than two categories** of response, the process is more complicated. If the categories can be assigned numerical codes on an interval scale , such that the difference between any two successive values can be interpreted in a constant fashion (eg the difference between 2 and 3, say, has the same meaning as the difference between 5 and 6), then this variable can be treated as a numerical variable for the purposes of multiple regression. The different categories of social class are usually treated in this way. If, on the other hand, the nominal qualitative variable has more than two categories, and the codes assigned to the different categories cannot be interpreted in an arithmetic framework, then handling this variable is more complex. $(k-1)$ binary dummy variables have to be created, where k is the number of categories of the nominal variable. A baseline category is chosen against which all of the other categories are compared; then each dummy variable that is created distinguishes one category of interest from the baseline category. Knowing how to code these dummy variables is not straightforward; details may be obtained from Armitage, Berry and Matthews (2001).[4]

A binary dependent variable — logistic regression

It is possible to formulate a linear model which relates a number of explanatory variables to a single *binary* dependent variable, such as treatment outcome, classified as success or failure. The right hand side of the equation defining the model is similar to that of the multiple linear regression equation. However, because the dependent variable (a dummy variable typically coded as 0 for failure and 1 for success) is not distributed Normally, and cannot be interpreted if its predicted value is not 0 or 1, multiple regression analysis cannot be sanctioned. Instead, a particular transformation is taken of the *probability*, *p*, of one of the two outcomes of the dependent variable (say, a success); this is called the **logistic** or **logit** transformation, where $\text{logit}(p) = \log_e[p/(1-p)]$. A special iterative process, called maximum likelihood, is then used to estimate the coefficients of the model instead of the ordinary least squares approach used in multiple regression. This results in an estimated **multiple linear logistic regression equation**, usually abbreviated to **logistic regression**, of the form:

$$\text{Logit } P = \log_e[P/(1-P)] = a + b_1x_1 + b_2x_2 + \ldots + b_kx_k$$

where *P* is the predicted value of *p*, the observed proportion of successes.

It is possible to perform significance tests on the coefficients of the logistic equation to determine which of the explanatory variables are important independent predictors of the outcome of interest, say 'success'. The estimated logistic regression coefficients, relevant confidence intervals, test statistics and *P*-values are usually contained in a table which is similar to that seen in a multiple regression output.

It is useful to note that the *exponential* of each coefficient is interpreted as the **odds ratio** of the outcome (eg success) when the value of the associated explanatory variable is increased by one, after adjusting for the other explanatory variables in the model. The odds ratio may be taken as an estimate of the **relative risk** if the probability of success is low. Odds ratios and relative risks are discussed in Chapter 2 — Research Designs 2. Thus, if a particular explanatory variable represents treatment (coded, for example, as 0 for the control treatment and 1 for a novel treatment), then the exponential of its coefficient in the logistic equation represents the *odds* or *relative* risk of success (say 'disease remission') for the novel treatment compared to the control treatment. A relative risk of one indicates that the two treatments are equally effective, whilst if its value is two, say, the risk of disease remission is twice as great on the novel treatment as it is on the control treatment.

The logistic model can also be used to predict the probability of success, say, for a particular individual whose values are known for all the explanatory variables. Furthermore, the percentages of individuals in the sample correctly predicted by the model as successes and failures can be shown in a classification table, as a way of assessing the extent to which the model can be used for prediction. Further details can be obtained in texts such as Kleinbaum (1994)[5] and Menard (1995).[6]

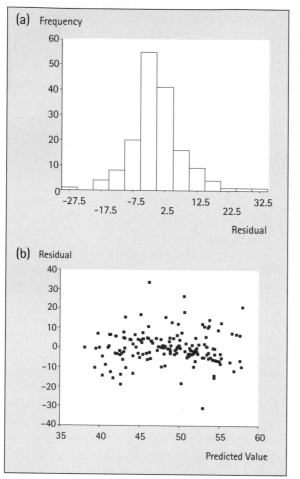

Fig. 2 Diagrams, using model residuals, for assessing the underlying assumptions in the multiple regression analysis

Checking the assumptions underlying a regression analysis

It is important, both in simple and multiple regression, to check the assumptions underlying the regression analysis in order to ensure that the model is valid. This stage is often overlooked as most statistical software does not do this automatically. The assumptions are most easily expressed in terms of the **residuals** which are determined by the computer program in the process of a regression analysis. The residual for each individual is the difference between his or her observed value of y and the corresponding fitted value, Y,

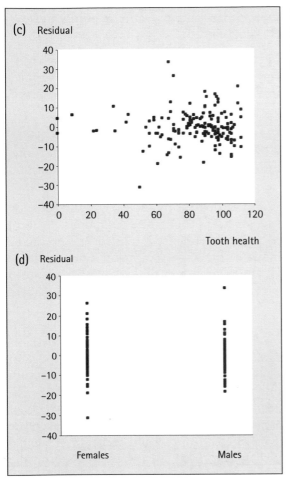

Fig. 2 (cont) Diagrams, using model residuals, for assessing the underlying assumptions in the multiple regression analysis

obtained from the model. The assumptions are listed in the following bullet points, and illustrated in the example at the end of the chapter:

- The residuals are Normally distributed. This is most easily verified by eyeballing a histogram of the residuals; this distribution should be symmetrical around a mean of zero (Fig. 2a).

- The residuals have constant variability for all the fitted values of y. This is most easily verified by plotting the residuals against the predicted values of *y*; the resulting plot should produce a random scatter of points and should not exhibit any funnel effect (Fig. 2b).

- The relationship between *y* and each of the explanatory variables (there is only one *x* in simple linear regression) is linear. This is most easily verified by plotting the residuals against the values of the explanatory variable; the resulting plot should produce a random scatter of points (Fig. 2c).

- The observations should be independent. This assumption is satisfied if each individual in the sample is represented only once (so that there is one point per individual in the scatter diagram in simple linear regression).

If all of the above assumptions are satisfied, the multiple regression equation can be investigated further. If there is concern about the assumptions, the most important of which are linearity and independence, a transformation can be taken of either *y* or of one or more of the *x*'s, or both, and a new multiple regression equation determined. The assumptions underlying this redefined model have to be verified before proceeding with the multiple regression analysis.

Example

A study assessed the impact of oral health on the life quality of patients attending a primary dental care practice, and identified the important predictors of their oral health related quality of life. The impact of oral health on life quality was assessed using the UK oral health related quality of life measure, obtained from a sixteen-item questionnaire covering aspects of physical, social and psychological health (McGrath *et al.*, 2000).[7] The data relate to a random sample of 161 patients selected from a multi-surgery NHS dental practice. Oral health quality of life score (OHQoL) was regressed on the explanatory variables shown in Table 2 with their relevant codings ('tooth health' is a composite indicator of dental health generated from attributing weights to the status of the tooth: 0 = missing, 1 = decayed, 2 = filled and 4 = sound).

The output obtained from the analysis includes an analysis of variance table (Table 1). The *F*-ratio obtained from this table equals 5·68, with 9 degrees of freedom in the numerator and 151 degrees of freedom in the denominator. The associated *P*-value, $P < 0.001$, indicates that there is substantial evidence to reject the null hypothesis that all the partial regression coefficients are equal to zero. Additional information from the output gives an adjusted $R^2 = 0.208$, indicating that approximately one fifth of the variability of OHQoL is explained by its linear relationship with the explanatory variables included in the model. This implies that approximately 80% of the variation is unexplained by the model.

Incorporating the estimated regression coefficients from Table 2 into an equation, gives the following estimated multiple regression model:

$$
\begin{aligned}
\text{OHQoL} = {} & 52 \cdot 58 - 2 \cdot 83 \text{gender} + 2 \cdot 97 \text{age} - \\
& 3 \cdot 28 \text{socialclass} - 5 \cdot 60 \text{toothache} - \\
& 2 \cdot 53 \text{brokenteeth} - 3 \cdot 08 \text{baddenture} - \\
& 1 \cdot 79 \text{sore} - 4 \cdot 02 \text{looseteeth} + 0 \cdot 079 \text{toothhealth}
\end{aligned}
$$

The estimated coefficients of the model can be interpreted in the following fashion, using both a binary variable (gender) and a numerical variable (tooth health) as examples:

OHQoL is 2·8 less for males, on average, than it is for females (ie it decreases by 2·8 when gender increases by one unit, going from females to males), after adjusting for the all the other explanatory variables in the model, and

OHQoL increases by 0·079 on average as the tooth health score increases by one unit, after adjusting for the all the other explanatory variables in the model.

It can be seen from Table 2 that the coefficients that are significantly different from zero, and therefore judged to be important independent predictors of OHQoL, are gender (males having a lower mean OHQoL score than females), social class (those in higher social classes having a higher mean OHQoL score), tooth health (those with a higher tooth health score having a higher mean OHQoL score), and having a toothache in the last year (those with toothache having a lower mean OHQoL score than those with no toothache). Whether or not the patient was older or younger than 55 years, had or did not have a poor denture, sore gums or loose teeth in the last year were not significant ($P > 0 \cdot 05$) independent predictors of OHQoL.

The four components, a, b, c and d, of Figure 2 are used to test the underlying assumptions of the model. In Figure 2a, it can be seen from the histogram of the residuals that their distribution is approximately Normal. When the residuals are plotted against the predicted (ie fitted) values of OHQoL (Fig. 2b), there is no tendency for the residuals to increase or decrease with increasing predicted values, indicating that the constant variance assumption is satisfied. It should be noted, furthermore, that the residuals are evenly scattered above and below zero, demonstrating that the mean of the residuals is zero. Figure 2c shows the residuals plotted against the numerical explanatory variable, tooth health. Since there is no systematic pattern for the residuals in this diagram, this suggests that the relationship between the two variables is linear. Finally, considering gender which is just one of the binary explanatory variables, it can be seen from Fig. 2d that the distribution of the residuals is fairly similar in males and females, suggesting that the model fits equally well in the two groups. In fact, similar patterns were seen for all the other explanatory variables, when the residuals were plotted against each of them. On the basis of these results, it can be concluded that the assumptions underlying the multiple regression analysis are satisfied.

A logistic regression analysis was also performed on this data set. The oral health quality of life score was scored as 'zero' in those individuals with values of it less than or equal to 42 (the median value in a 1999 national survey), and as 'one' if their values were greater than 42, the latter grouping comprising individuals believed to have an enhanced oral health related quality of life. The outcome variable in the logistic regression was then the logit of the proportion of individuals with an enhanced oral health quality of life; the explanatory variables were the same as those used in the multiple regression analysis. Having a toothache, a poorly fitting denture or loose teeth in the last year as well as being of a lower social class were the only variables which resulted in an odds ratio of enhanced oral health quality of life which was significantly less than one; no other coefficients in the model were significant. For example, the estimated coefficient in the logistic regression equation associated with toothache was -1.84 ($P < 0.001$); therefore, the estimated odds ratio for an enhanced oral health quality of life was its exponential equal to 0.16 (95% confidence interval 0.06 to 0.43). This suggests that the odds of an enhanced oral health quality of life was reduced by 84% in those suffering from a toothache in the last year compared to those not having a toothache, after taking all the other variables in the model into account.

It should be noted, however, that when the response variable is really quantitative, it is generally better to try to find an appropriate multiple regression equation rather than to dichotomise the values of y and fit a logistic regression model. The advantage of the logistic regression in this situation is that it may be easier to interpret the results of the analysis if the outcome can be considered a 'success' or a 'failure', but dichotomising the values of y will lose information; furthermore, the significance and values of the regression coefficients obtained from the logistic regression will depend on the arbitrarily chosen cut-off used to define 'success' and 'failure'.

The authors would like to thank Dr Colman McGrath for kindly providing the data for the example.

1   Bulman J S, Osborn J F. *Statistics in Dentistry*. London: British Dental Journal Books, 1989.
2   Chatterjee S, Price B. *Regression Analysis by Example*. 3rd edn. Chichester: Wiley, 1999.
3   Petrie A, Sabin C. *Medical Statistics at a Glance*. Oxford: Blackwell Science, 2000.
4   Armitage P, Berry G, Matthews, J N S. *Statistical Methods in Medical Research*. 4th edn. Oxford: Blackwell Scientific Publications, 2001.
5   Kleinbaum D G, Klein M. *Logistic Regression: a Self-Learning Text*. Heidelberg: Springer, 2002.
6   Menard S. *Applied Logistic Regression Analysis*. Sage University Paper series on Quantitative Applications in the Social Sciences, series no. 07-106. Town: Sage University Press, 1995.
7   McGrath C, Bedi R, Gilthorpe M S. Oral health related quality of life – views of the public in the United Kingdom. *Community Dent Health* 2000; 17: 3-7.

Repeated measures

7

Consider the situation in which there is a single quantitative variable of interest that is measured on each individual on several different occasions. Typically, these occasions are defined time points (usually including pre-treatment as well as various post-treatment times), so that each individual contributes a series of readings. The main objective of the study may be to compare the responses on this variable when each individual has been assigned to one of two or more treatments groups.

Consider, secondly, another situation that involves the periodontal treatment of a particular condition occurring at several sites within each patient's mouth. Suppose a trial of two or more treatments is undertaken and patients are randomly allocated to the treatment groups. Although observations, for example of pocket depth, are made before and after treatment at each site, the same treatment is given to all the sites in a given patient. The response at each site is then recorded as the change in pocket depth, so that each patient has one response from each of his pockets.

These two examples are similar in the sense that each patient produces several observations, but in the first example, the observations are ordered in time whereas in the second, the observations represent different sites measured at the same time and are thus not ordered.

Difficulties in interpreting this type of data arise because there are two sources of variability, both within- and between-patients. Within a patient, the observations differ because they are taken at different times or are obtained from different pockets, while if the mean value of the responses is calculated for each patient, these means will differ between patients.

In the analysis of such data, various strategies could be adopted. These are discussed in, for example, Everitt (1995)[1] and Matthews *et al.* (1990).[2] Some methods are relatively simple, but not 100% efficient; others may be more efficient but are much more complex and may require the use of very specialised computer programs; there are others which are simple but which are invalid and thus may yield totally misleading results.

Thus three strategies are:

1 Calculate the mean value (or some other single summary measure of the response, for example a regression coefficient) for each patient. The data set is now reduced to one observation from each of the patients who have been randomly allocated treatments. The methods of analysis are the conventional two-sample t-test or its non-parametric equivalent if there are two treatments, or one-way analysis of variance (ANOVA) or the Kruskal–Wallis test if there are three or more treatments. This method loses information about the variability of the observations within patients.

2 Perform an analysis which takes account of both sources of variation. The first example in which the observations are taken serially in time will have a more complex analysis than the second where the observations are merely repeated observations on the same individual.

3 Ignore the variability between patients, and pretend that all the observations are independent; that is, analyse 50 observations on one patient as though they were the same as one observation on each of 50 patients. This strategy may produce a significant result but is totally *invalid*.

Strategy 1. Use summary measures

This first approach is the one which is recommended for its simplicity and the fact that it is safe in the sense that the significance tests will tend to be conservative. This implies that if a result is statistically significant using this method, it will almost certainly be significant using even the most complicated statistical techniques. Details of this method are given here in the situation in which each patient receives a single treatment and the outcome variable is quantitative (although the method can be used for ordered qualitative data). All the information on each individual is reduced to just one single measure which is believed, in the context of the particular experiment, to be a useful summary of the responses. For example, it may be decided that for an individual patient, the mean of the responses at all the time points after the start of the treatment, or of all the sites within his or her mouth, is a sensible representation of the individual's overall response to treatment. The analysis is then restricted to this summary measure, and the summary measures are compared in the individuals in one treatment group with those in another group using a simple two-sample comparison, such as the two-sample *t*-test or the Mann-Whitney or Wilcoxon rank sum tests. If there are more than two treatment groups, it is possible to use the one-way ANOVA or the non-parametric Kruskal-Wallis test. Easy to understand, simple to execute and, fortunately, scientifically justifiable!

Often the choice of the summary measure is straightforward. However, on some occasions it may be difficult to know which single measure best describes the set of responses for an individual. The chosen measure must focus on the important issues and describe what is relevant in the particular investigation. In fact, if it is necessary to investigate different aspects of the response, the analysis may be repeated for two or more different summary measures.

In the context of the example of a clinical trial where observations are made at different points in time, two questions may be of interest: Are the responses on average higher (or lower) for treatment A than for treatment B? Alternatively, if the treatment were expected to change (consistently increase or decrease) the value of the response over the whole of the treatment period, it might be better to calculate the regression coefficient of the response on time, that is, the rate at which the response changes for each patient. It is important to realise that these two summary measures answer two different questions. In the first case, the analysis concentrates on the comparison of the mean level of response and totally ignores the rate at which the patients improve. In the second, the rate at which the patients improve is compared between the two treatments, totally ignoring the level of the responses. It is essential to choose the summary measure(s) *before* the study is conducted, thus ensuring that the choice cannot be influenced by the results, but this should be clear from the objectives and protocol.

In the periodontal disease example investigating change in pocket depth, there is a further complication in that the number of observations is unlikely to be the same for each patient; not all patients will have exactly the same number of gingival pockets. If the number of observations per patient varies very widely it may be more efficient to use a **weighted analysis** of the summary measure in order to take more account of the mean for a patient who has say 30 pockets than for a patient who has just one pocket. However, because the variability of the responses within patients will almost certainly be very much less than the variability of the means of the patients, there may not be a very great gain in efficiency as compared with the unweighted analysis.

Typical summary measures

The same summary measure is determined for every individual in the study. There are various summary measures that can be used. Some of the more usual ones in the context of the first time-related example are:

- The overall post-treatment mean of the responses for an individual.

- The difference between the initial and final responses. (This would correspond to the patient's mean change in pocket depth in the periodontal disease example).

- The percentage change between the initial and final responses.

- The maximum (or minimum) response.

- The time to reach the maximum (or minimum) value.

- The time to reach a particular value (eg some fixed percentage of the baseline value).

- The estimated slope of the linear regression line (provided a straight line relationship is appropriate). In this situation, it may be sensible to make adjustments in the analysis for the fact that some slope estimates may be more precise (ie have smaller standard errors) than others.

- The area under the curve.

Refinements on the basic procedure

The summary measure for the first time-related example may comprise one or more of the post-treatment responses, ignoring the pre-treatment value(s). However, the pre-treatment reading for each individual (or, if there is more than one pre-treatment reading for an individual, the mean of these pre-treatment readings) could be incorporated into the summary measure. For example, the summary measure might be the difference between the mean of the post-treatment responses and the pre-treatment value (ie the reading or the mean of the readings, as appropriate). Alternatively, instead of incorporating the pre-treatment value(s) into the measure itself, the power of the comparisons can be increased by using the **analysis of covariance**, with the pre-treatment value as the covariate, instead of the simple comparison of groups which makes no adjustment for the pre-treatment value.

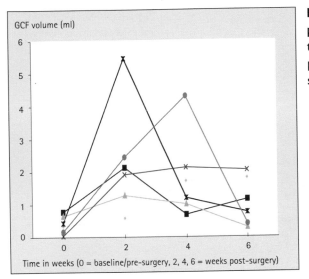

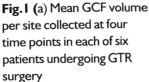

Fig. 1 (a) Mean GCF volume per site collected at four time points in each of six patients undergoing GTR surgery

Plotting the data

It is always helpful, if possible, to plot the data to give a broad indication of what is happening. In the first example, the raw data could be plotted against time. All the information could be retained in one diagram, so that every response for all individuals is shown. However, if there are a large number of individuals, this can produce a confusing diagram which fails to achieve its aim of demonstrating trends and relationships. In such instances, a separate diagram can be produced for each treatment group (Fig. 1a and Fig. 1b). Alternatively, separate graphs of the responses against time for each individual can be drawn; each should be drawn on the same scale, perhaps grouping the graphs for each treatment in a grid. Often there are so many graphs that it becomes unwieldy to include them all in a paper. Then, just representative examples which are believed to illustrate particular types of response structures may be included. The subjectivity of this approach may be open to criticism, so the choices should be justified.

It is tempting to produce average curves for each treatment group by plotting the mean (with confidence interval or standard error bars) of the responses at each time point against time. Although this is a simple approach to incorporate into a one diagram the information from many individuals, there is always the danger that the mean curve for a treatment group is not representative of any

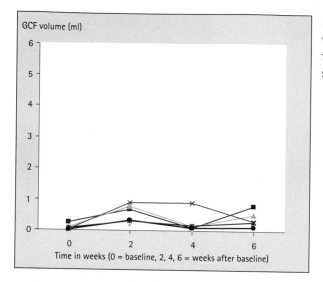

Fig. I (b) Mean GCF volume per site collected at four time points in each of six control patients

single individual's curve. Sometimes, depending on the quantity of the data, it is possible to show both the mean curve(s) and those for the individuals in a single graph, distinguishing the two by, for example, using a solid black line for the mean curve, and different pastel colours for the individuals.

If summary measures are used to analyse the data, it is often helpful to plot them. The distribution of the chosen summary measure should certainly be investigated by producing, separately for each treatment group, a diagram, such as a histogram or box-plot, of its values. The distribution will influence the choice of statistical test to compare values in the different treatment groups or may suggest that the data should be transformed. If the summary measures are not Normally distributed with approximately constant variance, a non-parametric method, such as the Wilcoxon rank sum test may be appropriate to compare these measures in the two treatment groups or the Kruskal–Wallis one-way ANOVA when there are more than two groups. Alternatively, a parametric analysis, such as the two-sample t-test or the one-way ANOVA, would be preferable for Normally distributed measures (or their transform). Sometimes, if more than one summary measure is investigated, it is useful to plot one summary measure against another. For example, the two summary measures might be minimum response and the time to reach that minimum response. The resulting scatter plot may provide insights which would not be available from the raw data alone.

Example

As an example, consider a small study (based on data kindly provided by Dr Gareth Griffiths and Dr Leyla Kuru of the Eastman Dental Institute for Oral Health Care Sciences, University College London) which was concerned with investigating the cellular activities involved in periodontal wound healing. Gingival crevicular fluid (GCF) accumulates in the gingival crevice and is considered to reflect ongoing cellular activities in the surrounding periodontal tissue. For each patient undergoing guided tissue regeneration (GTR) surgery, the volume of GCF was collected from 3–4 sites adjacent to the intrabony defects on molar teeth. The volume of GCF was also collected from 2–4 randomly chosen healthy molar sites in each patient in a control group not undergoing surgery. Samples were collected at baseline (pre-surgery) and then at 2, 4 and 6 weeks after baseline. The mean volume of GCF per site was determined from the total volume collected from each patient at each time point. The preliminary results from 12 patients are shown in Fig. 1a and Fig. 1b. The maximum of the mean GCF volume for each patient at a given time point in the 6-week period was used as a summary measure. These maxima were 1·81, 1·28, 2·14, 5·46, 4·31 and 2·12 µl in the surgery group, and 0·16, 0·81, 0·79, 0·91, 0·31 and 0·32 µl in the control group. The median of these maxima was 2·13 µl (range 1·28 to 5·46 µl) in the surgery group and 0·56 µl (range 0·16 to 0·91 µl) in the control group: the difference in medians was 1·57 µl. Since the sample size was very small (there were only six patients in each group) and it was therefore difficult to establish Normality, the non-parametric Wilcoxon rank sum test was used to compare the two groups of maxima; this gave $P = 0·002$, indicating that, on average, the maximum volume of GCF produced was greater in the surgical group.

Strategy 2. More complex analyses taking account of within- and between-patient variability

The data can be analysed using more complex **analysis of variance** (ANOVA) techniques. The analysis of variance covers a wide range of experimental designs. It is important to ensure that all the appropriate considerations relating to the analysis of variance model are taken into account in any particular design. In this situation, **repeated measures ANOVA**, available in the more sophisticated statistical software packages, can be used.

The use of repeated measures analysis of variance relies on being able to specify the model appropriately and understand its underlying assumptions, both of which present some difficulty to the novice statistician. Should fixed or random effects be specified in the model? Are the data Normally distributed? Is there sphericity or circularity of the covariance matrix? How should Mauchly's test be interpreted? What is the correction factor correcting? Should a multivariate approach be used? Do we need orthogonal polynomials to transform the variable? Are we able to interpret the ANOVA tables in the output? These are some of the questions to be answered if the repeated measures ANOVA approach to analysing this data is to be used. Clearly, it is not for everyone!

An added problem is that the design for a repeated measures ANOVA should be balanced. In the first time-related example, this requires that each individual should have the same number of measurements at equal time intervals. This may be reasonable in a well controlled experiment; a completely balanced design can be specified in which the same number of responses are measured at particular pre-determined time points for all individuals, recognising that there may be just a few missing observations because of factors which are beyond control (a transport strike, a bereavement in the family, etc). However, in some longitudinal studies, this may not be possible, and the data may be a series of readings on individuals at essentially random points in time. A repeated measures ANOVA on these data would have to ensure that there are complete data at specified time points, requiring many missing values at these times to be estimated and some existing values at other times to be ignored. This is an extremely inefficient approach to the analysis and is not to be recommended.

Even more **complex models** can be used, which take into account the fact that the time points at which measurements are made for different individuals may vary, and which allow for missing observations. For example, a suitable regression-type model might be specified and maximum likelihood used, instead of ordinary least squares, to estimate its parameters and standard errors. This approach is not simple, relies on the assumptions underlying the model being satisfied, and is best left to the experienced statistician.

Similarly, the *multilevel modelling* approach (Leyland and Goldstein, 2001)[3] is appropriate but requires considerable expertise and dedicated software (eg MLwiN: information on www.ioe.ac.uk/MLwiN) to execute. In multilevel modelling, the hierarchical (or nested) structure of the data is taken into account. When there are repeated measures, such as in the examples quoted, the hierarchy consists of times or sites within individuals. A regression model is specified with two 'levels', the lower level representing times/ sites and the upper level representing individuals. A covariate is included in the model to represent the treatment effect and additional covariates can also be included to represent the effects of other factors such as gender and age. The multilevel model incorporates random residuals which vary between the units at each level, and uses generalised least squares (rather than ordinary least squares as in straightforward regression) to estimate the parameters of interest.

Strategy 3. How not to proceed

One method that should not be attempted in the time-related example is to compare the groups at each time point, using, for two groups, a two-sample t-test or a non-parametric equivalent, such as the Wilcoxon rank sum test. There are a number of reasons why this is inadvisable:

- The within-patient changes over time are ignored.

- The successive tests are not independent.

- The whole process may involve many significance tests, thereby increasing the probability of the Type I error.

- It may be difficult to come to some overall conclusion about the difference between groups, and impossible to obtain a single estimate of this difference.

A second, even worse method is to classify all the observations only according to the treatments and pretend that the observations in each treatment group are independent; that is to take no account of the patients and the variability within patients. This may well lead to an apparent significant difference between the treatments but, because it ignores an important source of variability, will lead to a totally invalid result.

Discussion

This chapter has reviewed some methods of analysis to be used when there are repeated observations on the same study unit; in the case of the examples

Table I Results of three methods of analysis of a trial of the effect of three mouth washing solutions on gingival pockets (Abstracted from Osborn, 1987)[5]

	Metronidazole	Quinine sulphate	Saline
Number of patients	9	5	5
Total number of pockets per treatment group	263	145	139
Number of pockets per patient (range)	21 to 49	24 to 41	19 to 40
Mean reduction in pocket depth per patient (mm)	1·0288	0·7235	0·5905
SE(mean) (mm) simple summary measure method	0·2066	0·2772	0·2772
SE(mean) (mm) weighted summary measure method	0·2061	0·2762	0·2774
SE(mean) (mm) ignoring patients (invalid method)	0·0705	0·0949	0·0970

described, the study unit is the individual patient. However the problem is much more general and data are often analysed without taking account of the structure of the raw data. A very common error is to design a multi-centre study, perhaps because any one centre cannot generate sufficient patients, but to do the analysis pretending that the results are from a single centre, thus ignoring the big differences that almost always exist between centres. The error can be even worse in a large international multi-centre study, in which say, Great Britain is represented by a single clinic in North Wales. It is exceedingly important that multi-centre studies are analysed as multi-centred and not as though the data are generated by a random sample of patients from, say, Europe.

This problem has been recognised in periodontal research for some time and earlier papers on the subject are Blomqvist (1985)[4] and Osborn (1987).[5] Both papers investigate the multiple site per patient example. Blomqvist suggests that the simple summary method be used, the summary measure being the mean change in pocket depth for each patient. On the other hand, Osborn compares Blomqvist's method with a weighted summary measure method (that is, taking account of the number of observations on each patient and the variability of the observations within each patient), and also the invalid method which assumes that all the observations in each treatment group are independent. The data were from a small trial to compare three mouth washing solutions (containing metronidazole, quinine sulphate or saline solution) for the treatment of gingival pockets. Some of the results of the comparison of the methods of analysis are shown in Table 1. It can be seen that the weighted analysis, which is much more complicated than the simple summary method, produces practically identical values of the standard errors of the estimated treatment effects. There are clearly no statistically significant differences between the treatments if either of the two valid methods of analysis is done. In contrast, the differences are highly significant according to the mistaken analysis. The analysis of a repeated measures study must be based on the number of subjects, not only on the total number of observations.

1   Everitt B S. The analysis of repeated measures: a practical review with examples *The Statistician* 1995; 44: 113–135.
2   Matthews J N S, Altman D G, Campbell M J, Royston P. Analysis of serial measurements in medical research. Br Med J 1990; 300: 230–235.
3   Leyland A H, Goldstein H. (eds) *Multilevel Modelling of Health Statistics*. Chichester: John Wiley and Sons, 2001.
4   Blomqvist N. On the choice of computational unit in statistical analysis. *J Clin Periodontol* 1985; 12: 873–876.
5   Osborn J. The choice of computational unit in the statistical analysis of unbalanced clinical trials. *J Clin Periodontol* 1987; 14: 519–523.

Systematic reviews and meta-analyses

8

A **systematic review** of research evidence is an efficient approach to integrating existing information, invariably a multiplicity of published articles, with a view to establishing whether the scientific findings are consistent. If so, it may be possible to draw conclusions and make recommendations about treatment regimens or observed effects which have greater credence than those obtained from individual studies. The systematic review relies on a specified checklist which determines which articles should be included in the review, and how each should be critically appraised to provide relevant information relating to the focus of the review.

Systematic reviews

The report of a systematic review is somewhat like that of a research paper; it contains a clear description of the aims, and the material and methods used by the reviewer. The alternative haphazard non-systematic review has no defined rules concerning the process of digesting the mass of information, and is open to abuse.

A systematic review serves various purposes:

- It reduces a large amount of information to a manageable size. This information can be assimilated quickly by healthcare providers, researchers and policy makers. At the initial stage, the systematic review distinguishes between those studies that are essentially unsound and those that provide useful and scientifically worthwhile results in relation to the question of interest.

- By combining the results from various studies which may have been conducted in slightly varying circumstances (eg using different definitions of disease or patient eligibility criteria), it may be possible to determine from the systematic review whether the results are consistent from study to study, and to generalise the results. Furthermore, a systematic review may offer the opportunity to explain any inconsistencies.

- It is usually cheaper and quicker to conduct a systematic review than to embark on a new study.

- It may reduce the delay between research discoveries and the implementation of new effective treatment strategies.

- The systematic review combines information from individual studies so that its overall sample size is greater than that of any one study, and this leads to an increase in the power of the investigation. Thus, the systematic review has a greater chance of eliciting significant treatment effects, which is particularly helpful if the prevalence of the condition is low or if the effect of interest if small.

- The systematic review has an increased sample size compared with any individual study so the estimates of the effects of interest are obtained with increased precision.

- A systematic review limits bias and improves the reliability and accuracy of recommendations because of its formalised and thorough method of investigation.

The **Cochrane Collaboration** (www.update-software.com/ccweb/cochrane/general.htm) is an international network of individuals and institutions which prepares systematic reviews of randomised controlled studies and of observational evidence. It helps to promote the development of systematic reviews by setting explicit standards for them. It provides a framework within which scientists of like interests can collaborate, and through its publication, the *Cochrane Database of Systematic Reviews*, allows electronic access to the latest detailed and highly structured reports on subjects of interest.

Meta-analysis

A special form of systematic review is a **meta-analysis** (sometimes called an overview); this is a statistical approach to combining the results from separate but similar studies to provide an overall *quantitative* summary of the effect of interest. A meta-analysis is thus a statistical analysis of a collection of statistical analyses from individual studies. Full details of the theory of meta-analysis may be obtained in Hedges and Olkin (1985).[1] In addition, a paper by Song et al. (1997)[2] provides a useful discussion of how to handle discrepancies in recommendations arising from different meta-analyses of what appear to be the same research question.

In principle, a meta-analysis proffers the advantages of increased power, and increased precision of its estimates, when compared with a single study. In practice, the meta-analysis is open to criticism, essentially on four grounds (Glass *et al.*, 1981):[3]

1 Because journals rarely publish studies in which the findings are non-significant, published research is biased in favour of significant results. A trial with a significant result is sometimes called a *positive* trial; a *negative* trial is one in which a clinically significant effect is essentially ruled out. This **publication bias** leads to biased meta-analysis results unless the meta-analyst makes a serious attempt to identify and use the results in books, dissertations, unpublished papers presented at professional meetings or located in retrieval systems for unpublished papers (such as SIGLE produced by the European Association for Grey Literature), etc.

2 The studies included in the meta-analysis may differ in respect of features such as design, outcome measure, measuring technique, definition of variables and subjects, and duration of follow-up. Such **clinical heterogeneity** needs to be explored carefully as it may affect the overall conclusions and the clinical implications of the review. Generally, a meta-analysis of clinical trials is restricted to include only those trials that are *randomised*. Additional requirements of blind or objective assessment of response, ideally with analysis by intention-to-treat and complete follow-up, are sometimes imposed (Peto, 1987).[4] Such trials are less likely to lead to biased results than those which do not possess these attributes.

3 The studies included in the meta-analysis may vary in their quality, and it has been shown (Jahad, 1996)[5] that a meta-analysis which comprises studies of high quality, as opposed to poor quality, tends to be less enthusiastic about an intervention. However, it can be argued that poorly designed or 'bad' studies should be included in the meta-analysis because of the inclusiveness of the method and the subjective nature of the considerations which might lead to their exclusion. The problem of including both 'good' and 'bad' studies can be handled empirically by conducting separate analyses for groups of studies of similar quality, and examining whether the results differ for poorly and well designed

studies. Sometimes, the results from all the studies are combined by assigning weights to the studies according to their relative quality, but this approach can be criticised on grounds of the arbitrariness of the assignment.

4 The results included in the meta-analysis may not be independent. This situation arises when a multivariate study provides more than one test of significance relevant to the hypothesis that the meta-analysis is examining. Also, non-independence of the results may arise when the studies are conducted by the same investigator at different times, or by different investigators who have communicated with each other and modified their studies on the basis of earlier results. Furthermore, some trials are published more than once.

Example

Meta-analyses in dentistry are not very common. The example used in this chapter, a meta-analysis by van Rijkom *et al.* (1998),[6] can be criticised but is, nevertheless, thorough and accessible. The authors used a meta-analysis to estimate the overall caries inhibiting effect of fluoride gels applied to the permanent teeth of children aged 6 to 15 years. Each of the 19 studies included in the analysis, referenced by study number at the end of this chapter, was obtained from a MEDLINE search of the published literature of English and German studies. All these studies satisfied various selection inclusion and exclusion criteria, and their follow-up periods were between 1·5 and 3 years (median 3 years). In particular, each of the chosen studies was a randomised controlled trial in which the effect of the fluoride gel treatment was compared with no treatment or placebo treatment. In fact, some of the 19 studies were independent substudies of a larger study which had been split into two to reflect differences in general fluoride regimen. The inhibiting effect of the treatment was expressed for each study by the prevented fraction (PF); this was calculated as the difference in the incidence between the decayed, missing and filled surfaces (DMFS) in the control group (lc) and the incidence in the experimental group (le), divided by that in the control group [ie $PF = (lc - le)/lc$]. The absolute difference between the incidences in the two groups was standardized (ie divided by lc) since the PF was assumed to be less sensitive to experimental circumstances, such as the age range of the study population and the duration of the study, than (lc – le).

The effect of interest in a meta-analysis

Explaining the effect of interest

Suppose that the meta-analysis comprises k studies, and that θ_i denotes the value of an appropriate measure of the **effect of interest** in the ith study. In a clinical trial, this will usually be the effect of the experimental treatment relative to the control treatment. If the outcome variable is quantitative, θ_i is typically the difference between the experimental and control treatment means in the population or some standardized version of this difference. If the outcome is binary, for example 'success' or 'failure', θ_i is often the logarithm of the odds ratio or relative risk. In the fluoride gel example, the effect of interest is the prevented fraction (PF), expressed as a percentage.

There are two approaches to combining the information in a meta-analysis. The **parametric approach** is usually adopted; this assumes that the effect of interest in each study is Normally distributed. Note that both the difference between the means and its standardized difference are Normally distributed for Normally distributed data; similarly, the logarithm of the relative risk, equal to the difference in the logarithms of the two risks, is approximately Normally distributed. The PF in this example is assumed to be approximated Normally distributed. The parametric approach focuses on combining the results from the k studies, estimating the overall effect of interest, with its confidence interval, testing its significance and interpreting these results. Occasionally, a **non-parametric approach** is used which makes no distributional assumptions about the effect of interest. However, the non-parametric methods often require the raw data from each study, which can limit their use, and they are not described here.

Displaying the effect of interest

Initially, it is helpful to **display** the quantitative results from each study both in tabular and diagrammatic form. The table includes the relevant information on each trial; for example, the sample size, baseline patient characteristics, information on inclusion criteria and withdrawal rates, and the effects of interest, such as the odds ratio. Table 1 summarises some of the more important features of the selected studies in the fluoride gel example.

Table I Summary of study results arranged according to application method and

Study no[§]	Fluoride regimen[*]	Applic. Freq. Times/year	Method[†]	Control group		
				Incident DMFS	SEM	n
1	1	1	1	7·26	0·46	10
2	2	1	1	3·82	0·29	31
3	2	1	1	8·61	0·61	17
4	1	1	1	2·15	0·17	17
5	2	1	1	1·91	0·17	15
6	2	2	1	7·19	0·32	31
7	1	2	1	8·52	0·37	31
8	2	2	1	8·15	0·87	7
9	2	2	1	4·40	0·38	10
10	1	2	1	3·24	0·22	20
11	2	4	1	4·21	0·32	16
12	1	90	1	2·20	0·20	22
13	1	6	2	4·26	0·37	14
14	1	30	2	4·40	0·42	5
15	2	30	2	3·44	0·38	4
16	1	360	3	6·86	0·37	24
17	1	360	3	8·34	0·28	44
18	1	360	3	7·70	0·29	38
19	1	360	3	6·39	0·23	41

*Fluoride regimen: 1 = assumed non-fluoride toothpaste,
 2 = assumed fluoride toothpaste or non-fluoride toothpaste including fluoride water
†Method: 1 = tray > 1%, 2 = brush > 1%, 3 = brush < 1%
‡n: study size §These study numbers are referenced at the end of the chapter

The most usual pictorial representation (Fig. 1) is sometimes called a 'forest plot'. It shows the estimated effect of interest (in the fluoride gel example it is the PF but might, in other circumstances, be the standardized difference in means or the odds ratio) for each of the separate studies in the meta-analysis. The confidence intervals for the true effect in each case, as well as the overall estimated effect (and related confidence interval) from the pooled data from all the studies, are also indicated. An explanation of the method used to calculate the overall estimated effect is given in the section entitled 'calculating

plication frequency[6]				
Experimental group			PF (%)	95% CI (%)
cident DMFS	SEM	$n^{\ddagger}$		
5·46	0·44	103	37	23 to 52
3·14	0·23	278	18	0 to 35
6·51	0·50	182	24	9 to 40
2·07	0·20	148	4	–20 to 28
1·83	0·20	163	4	–23 to 31
6·68	0·32	296	7	–5 to 19
7·39	0·32	315	13	3 to 24
5·28	0·66	115	35	14 to 57
3·08	0·37	108	30	9 to 51
2·94	0·21	224	9	–8 to 27
2·74	0·26	145	35	19 to 51
1·57	0·16	337	29	9 to 48
3·94	0·35	161	8	–15 to 30
2·63	0·32	63	40	22 to 59
2·18	0·38	38	37	11 to 63
5·40	0·34	253	21	8 to 34
6·60	0·24	451	21	13 to 29
6·94	0·27	378	10	0 to 20
4·56	0·22	460	29	20 to 37

the effect of interest'. A vertical line, known as the 'line of no effect', is sometimes drawn in the diagram. It represents equal effectiveness of the treatments (for example, it would correspond to a value of zero for PF or a difference in means, or unity if the effect of interest were the odds ratio). In the fluoride gel example, only five of the confidence intervals for the true PFs cross the line of no effect, whereas twelve of the confidence intervals are to the right of it; this suggests that fluoride gel is an effective inhibitor of caries.

It is possible to get some idea of whether the estimates of the effects from

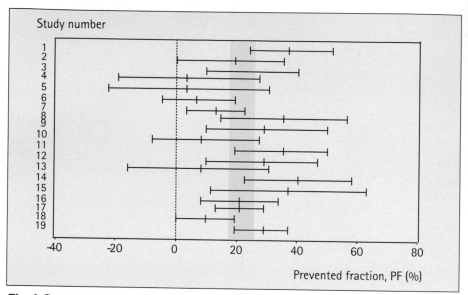

Fig. 1 Caries-inhibiting effect of fluoride gel treatment (PF with 95% confidence intervals) in 19 studies. The shaded area shows the 95% confidence interval for the pooled PF.[6]

the different studies are compatible by 'eye-balling' the forest plot. If the confidence intervals of the effects overlap, then the trials are likely to be compatible, whereas if there is no overlap, then they are incompatible. The confidence intervals in Fig. 1 show considerable overlap, suggesting that the results of the different studies are likely to be compatible. However, it should be noted that the estimated PFs show substantial variation, so this conclusion should be viewed with caution.

Checking for compatibility between the trials

A more formal approach to determining incompatibility is to perform a statistical test, described in detail in the section entitled 'Testing for homogeneity'. If, on the basis of the test result, the observed effects are more disperse than would be expected on the basis of chance alone, **statistical heterogeneity** is said to be present, ie the estimated effects exhibit considerable variation and are incompatible. Statistical heterogeneity may be caused by clinical heterogeneity, methodological differences or it may be related to unknown trial characteristics. The presence of statistical heterogeneity is indicated if the test of statistical *homogeneity* (homogeneity implies that the effects are equal) is significant. If the test is not significant, this does not imply that there must be statistical homogeneity. A non-significant result implies only that there is no evidence to reject the null hypothesis of homogeneity, and not that there is evidence to accept it. It should be pointed out that the test of statistical homogeneity has low power and, therefore, may fail to produce a statistically significant result unless there is marked heterogeneity. Whether or not the test is significant, it is important to provide an estimate of the extent to which there is statistical heterogeneity. Then, if this estimate indicates that there might be substantial statistical heterogeneity, the aspects of clinical heterogeneity which may be causing it should be investigated.

Calculating the effect of interest
The **overall estimate of effect** is usually taken as a weighted average of the estimates from the k individual studies in the meta-analysis. Thus the estimate of the overall effect is:

$$\hat{\theta} = \frac{\Sigma \hat{\theta}_i w_i}{\Sigma w_i}$$

where $\hat{\theta}_i$ is the estimated effect and w_i the weight of the ith study, and the sums extend over all k studies. Usually the weights are chosen to be inversely related to the variances of the estimated effects and this is approximately the same as choosing weights which are proportional to the sample size, so that the larger studies are given more weight than the smaller ones.

- A **fixed-effects** estimation method can be used if there is no evidence of statistical heterogeneity and/or if the meta-analysis comprises only a small number of studies. This approach assumes that the separate studies are the only ones that are of interest, and that the underlying true effect in each study is the same and equal to θ, ie $\theta_1 = \theta_2 = \ldots = \theta_k = \theta$. The variance of the estimated effect in each study comprises only the random variation in that study. When estimating the assumed common effect, θ, the weight attached to each θ_i is the reciprocal of its variance, so that more weight is given to the more precise estimate (ie that with a narrower confidence interval).

• If statistical heterogeneity is believed to be present, the **random-effects** estimation method may be appropriate. This approach assumes that the k separate studies are a random sample from a larger population of studies, and there is a population effect of interest, θ, about which the effects of the individual studies vary. Then $\hat{\theta}$ is an estimate of θ which is now the mean of the effects of interest obtained from all the studies in the population. As in the fixed-effects method, the weight for the ith study using the random-effects method is chosen to be the reciprocal of the variance of the estimated effect for that study. However, unlike the fixed-effects method, the random-effects method incorporates both the random variation within the study and the heterogeneity between the different studies into this variance. It produces a wider confidence interval for the overall estimate than the fixed-effects method, as would be expected from an estimate that reflects the heterogeneity of the estimates. It is important to remember that if there is statistical heterogeneity, caution must be adopted when interpreting the overall estimate of effect, however it is derived, and the reasons for the heterogeneity should be investigated.

Note that for both the fixed-effects and random-effects approaches, an approximate 95% **confidence interval** for the overall estimate of effect, θ, is given by $\hat{\theta} \pm 1 \cdot 96 \sqrt{(1/\Sigma \ w_i)}$. The w_i is the reciprocal of the variance of the estimated effect in the ith study. It is a measure of the random variation within the study for the fixed-effects approach, but includes the variation between the k estimated effects as well for the random-effects approach.

The authors in the fluoride gel example used two approaches to investigate heterogeneity. Firstly, they believed that the large overlap in the confidence intervals in the forest plot was an indication that there was no evidence of statistical heterogeneity. However, although there was considerable overlap in the confidence intervals, the estimates from the different studies showed substantial variation. Secondly, they used a multiple regression analysis to determine whether there were factors influencing the caries-inhibiting effect of fluoride gel application. This analysis showed no significant influence of the covariables that were thought could be relevant, namely, 'application frequency', 'application methods' (tray/brush), 'baseline caries prevalence' and 'general fluoride regimen'. Thus, they concluded that all studies could be regarded as equally effective, and the overall effect could be estimated using a fixed effects model. The weight for each study was chosen to be the inverse of the variance of the prevented fraction, PF; this gave an estimated overall PF of 22%. The 95% confidence interval for the true PF was 18% to 25%, the shaded area in Fig. 1; this excludes zero and suggests that fluoride gel was an effective inhibitor of caries in children of this age.

Hypothesis tests in meta-analysis

There are two hypothesis tests that are of crucial importance in a meta-analysis, one which tests for homogeneity of the effects of interest and the other which tests the significance of the overall treatment effect.

Testing for homogeneity

The test of the null hypothesis that the studies are homogenous with respect to their effects of interest should be performed initially, rather than relying solely on the subjective opinion obtained from the forest plot. The test of this hypothesis, sometimes called that of 'combinability', is usually based on the magnitude of the test statistic

$$Q = \Sigma\, w_i(\hat{\theta}_i - \hat{\theta})^2$$

which is assumed to follow a chi-squared distribution with $(k-1)$ degrees of freedom. As homogeneity is assumed under the null hypothesis in this test, the fixed-effects and the random-effects approaches are not distinguished, and the weight, w_i, is the same as that used in the fixed-effects approach, ie it is the reciprocal of the variance of the effect in the ith study ($i = 1, 2, 3, \ldots, k$), where that variance is a measure only of the random variation within the study.

It is interesting to note that, even though the confidence intervals for the PF's from the separate studies overlap (Fig. 1), the chi-squared test of homogeneity in the fluoride gel example gives a result which is marginally significant at the 5% level. This, together with the view that the different studies have estimated PFs which show considerable variation, should perhaps be an indication that combining the estimates of PF is questionable and that the overall estimate of the PF should be interpreted with caution.

In addition to the overall test which investigates heterogeneity (in fact, it tests homogeneity), it is possible to test for *funnel plot asymmetry* which assesses bias. Details may be obtained from Eggar *et al.,* (1997).[7] A **funnel plot** (Fig. 2) is a scatter plot of the sample size against the treatment effect estimate generated

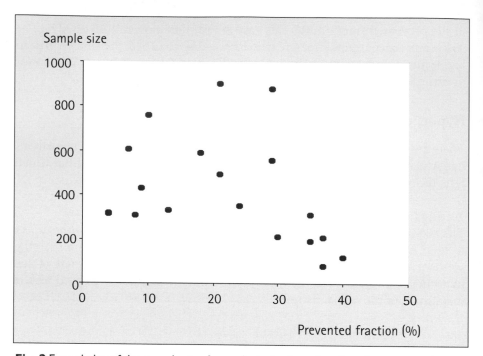

Fig. 2 Funnel plot of the sample size for each study plotted against the estimated prevented fraction, PF (%) for the 19 studies included in the meta-analysis

in an individual study. The sample size can be replaced by the precision of the estimated effect. Since the precision of the estimated treatment effect increases as the sample size of the component study increases, the results from small studies would be expected to show a wide scatter at the bottom of the graph, with the spread decreasing (narrowing to produce a funnel effect) at the top of the graph for the larger studies. The funnel plot will often be skewed and asymmetrical if bias is present, as demonstrated in Fig. 2. The lower left corner of the funnel is somewhat empty (ie lacking publications), indicating that some studies on small sample sizes with small effects are probably missing. The effect of this publication bias on the overall PF, however, is likely to be marginal, because the weight of such unpublished low-power studies is small. It is possible to measure the degree of asymmetry in a funnel plot, but the approach is of limited value if only a few trials are included (remembering that the unit of analysis is the randomised trial and not its patients).

Testing the treatment effect

The null hypothesis that the true effect of interest is zero (ie $H_0: \theta_1 = \theta_2 = \ldots = \theta_k = 0$ in the fixed-effects method, or $H_0: \theta = 0$ in the random-effects method) is tested using the test statistic:

$$U = \frac{(\Sigma \hat{\theta}_i w_i)}{\Sigma w_i}$$

which follows the chi-squared distribution with one degree of freedom. Each w_i is the reciprocal of the variance of the estimated effect of the ith study. In the fixed-effects approach, this variance is a measure only of the random variation within the study; in the random-effects method, the variance comprises both the random variation within the study and the variation between the estimated effects in the k studies. The test for the overall PF in the fluoride gel example gives a highly significant result ($P < 0.001$) indicating that the overall effect, estimated by a PF of 22% (95% confidence interval equal to 18% to 25%), is significantly different from zero. This implies that the fluoride gel is an effective inhibitor of caries in children of this age. Note that, as observed previously, zero lies outside the 95% confidence interval for the overall PF, as expected if the test result is significant.

The authors would like to thank Dr James Lewsey for his comments on earlier drafts of the manuscript.

1   Hedges L V, Olkin I. *Statistical Methods for Meta-analysis*. Academic Press: New York, 1985.
2   Song F, Landes D P, Glenny A-M, Sheldon T A. Prophylactic removal of impacted third molars: an assessment of published reviews. *Br Dent J* 1997; 182: 339-346.
3   Glass G, McGaw B, Smith M J. *Meta-analysis in Social Research*. Beverly Hills CA: Sage, 1981.
4   Peto R. Why do we need systematic overviews of randomised trials? *Stat Med* 1987; 6: 233-240.
5. Jahad A R, McQuay H J. Meta analyses to evaluate analgesic interventions: a systematic qualitative review of their methodology. *J Clin Epidemiol* 1996; 49: 235-243.
6. van Rijkom H M, Truin G J, van't Hof M A. A meta-analysis of clinical studies on the caries-inhibiting effect of fluoride gel treatment. *Caries Res* 1998; 32: 83-92.
7. Eggar M, Davey Smith G, Schneider M, Minder C. Bias in meta-analysis detected by a simple, graphical test. *Br Med J* 1997; 315: 629-634.

Studies, labelled by study number, included in the meta-analysis of van Rijkom et al. (1998)

1. Bryan F T, Williams J E. The cariostatic effectiveness of a phosphate-fluoride gel administered annually to school children: final results. *J Public Health Dent* 1970; **30:** 13-16.

2. Cons N C, Janerich D T, Senning R S. Albany topical fluoride study. *JADA* 1970; **2:** 263-266.

3. Horowitz H S, Doyle J. The effect on dental caries of topical applied acidulated phosphate-fluoride: Results after three years. *JADA* 1971; **82:** 359-365.

4. Szwejda L F. Fluorides in community programs: Results after two years from a fluoride gel applied topically. *J Public Health Dent* 1971; **31:** 241-242.

5. Szwejda L F. Fluorides in community programs:A study of four years of various fluorides applied topically to the teeth of children in fluoridated communities. *J Public Health Dent* 1972; **32:** 25-31.

6. Mainwaring P J, Naylor M N. A three-year clinical study to determine the separate and combined caries-inhibiting effects of sodium monofluoro-phosphate toothpaste and an acidulated phosphate-fluoride gel. *Caries Res* 1978; **12:** 202-212 (Sub-study with non-fluoride toothpaste).

7. Mainwaring P J, Naylor M N. A three-year clinical study to determine the separate and combined caries-inhibiting effects of sodium monofluoro-phosphate toothpaste and an acidulated phosphate-fluoride gel. *Caries Res* 1978; **12:** 202-212 (Sub-study with fluoride toothpaste).

8. Cobb H B, Rozier R G, Bawden J W. A clinical study of the caries preventive effects of a an APF solution and an APF thixotropic gel. *Pediatr Dent* 1980; **2:** 263-266.

9. Hagan P P, Bawden J W. The caries-preventive effects of full- and half-strength topical and acidulated phosphate fluoride. *Pediatr Dent* 1985; **7:** 185-191.

10. Olivier M, Brodeur J-M, Simard P L. Efficacy of APF treatments without prior toothcleaning targeted to high-risk children. *Community Dent Oral Epidemiol* 1992; **20:** 38-42.

11. Trubman G J, Crellin J A. Effect on dental caries of self-application of acidulated phosphate fluoride paste and gel. *JADA* 1973; **86:** 153-157.

12. Englander H R, Sherrill L T, Miller B G, Carlos J P, Mellberg J R, Senning R S. Incremental rates of dental caries after repeated topical sodium fluoride applications in children with lifelong consumption of fluoridated water. *JADA* 1971; **82:** 354-358.

13. Heifeetz S B, Horowitz H S, Driskoll W S. Two-year evaluation of a self-administered procedure for the topical application of acidulated phosphate-fluoride: Final report. *J Public Health Dent* 1970; **30:** 7-12.

14. Marthaler T M, König K G, Mühlemann H R. The effect of a fluoride gel usef for supervised tooth-brushing 15 or 30 times per year. *Helv Odont Acta* 1970; **14:** 67-77 (Sub-study with non-fluoride toothpaste).

15. Marthaler T M, König K G, Mühlemann H R. The effect of a fluoride gel usef for supervised tooth-brushing 15 or 30 times per year. *Helv Odont Acta* 1970; **14:** 67-77 (Sub-study with fluoride toothpaste).

16. Howat A P, Holloway P .J, Davies T G H. Caries prevention by daily supervised use of a MPF gel dentifrice. *Br J Dent* 1978; **145:** 233-235

17. Fogels H R, Alman J E, Meade I J, O'Donnell J P. The relative caries-inhibiting effects of a stannous fluoride dentifrice in a silica gel base. *JADA* 1979; **99:** 456-459.

18. Abrams R G, Chambers D W. Caries-inhibiting effect of a stannous fluoride silica gel dentifrice: A three-year clinical study. *Clin Prev Dent* 1980; **2:** 22-27.

19. Rule J T, Smith M R, Truelove R B, Macko D J, Castaldi C D. Caries inhibition of a dentifrice containing 0.78% sodium monofluorophosphate ion in a silica base. *Community Dent Oral Epidemiol* 1984; **12:** 213-217.

Bayesian statistics

9

Statistics can be defined as the *methods used to assimilate data, so that guidance can be given, and conclusions drawn, in situations which involve uncertainty*. In particular, **statistical inference** is concerned with drawing conclusions about particular aspects of a *population* when that population cannot be studied in full. Uncertainty arises here because the totality of the information is not available. Instead, to make inferences about the population, it is necessary to rely on a *sample* of data which is selected from the population; this sample data may be augmented, in certain circumstances, by auxiliary information which is obtained independently of the sample data. Clearly, uncertainty lies at the heart of statistics and statistical inference. This uncertainty is measured by a **probability** which therefore forms the crux of statistics and must be properly understood in order to interpret a statistical analysis.

Understanding statistics and probability

Measuring probability
A probability is a number that takes some value equal to or between zero and one. If the probability of the 'event' of interest is zero, then the event *cannot* occur. So, for example, the probability of drawing an 'eleven' from a pack of cards is zero because there is no such card. If the probability of the event of interest is unity, then the event *must* occur. Most probabilities lie somewhere between the two extremes; the closer the probability is to one, the more likely the event, the closer it is to zero, the less likely the event.

Defining probability
To take a particular example, suppose it is of interest to determine the probability that a man has a DMFT of zero (the event of interest). What is really meant by 'probability' in this setting? There are various ways of understanding a probability, the three most common being based on the following interpretations:

1. **Frequency.** This view of probability, also called *frequentist* or *empirical* probability, forms the basis for what is termed the *frequentist* or *classical* approach to statistical inference. The probability is defined only in situations or 'experiments' which can (at least, theoretically) be repeated again and again in essentially the same circumstances, under the constraint that the result from any one experiment is independent of any other. Therefore, it cannot be applied to a 'one-off' event, such as assessing the probability that Prince Charles will be king. Strictly, although every event is one-off, many events can be regarded as similar enough to satisfy the criteria laid down by the frequentist approach. The frequency definition of probability is then the *proportion* of times the event of interest occurs when the 'experiment' is repeated on many occasions, and is equivalent to a *relative frequency*. The frequency definition of probability is easily understood in the context of coin tossing, when a single toss of the coin can be regarded as the experiment and obtaining a 'head' as the event of interest. If a fair coin were tossed 1,000,000 times (that is, a large number of times), the 'frequency' interpretation of the probability of a head would be the number of heads obtained divided by 1,000,000, ie the proportion of heads. In the DMFT example, if there are 1,000 men in the population, then each man is regarded as the experiment, and a DMFT of zero is regarded as the event of interest. The probability that a man has a DMFT of zero is the proportion of the 1,000 men with a DMFT of zero.

2. **Subjective.** This view of probability, central to *Bayesian* inference, is also termed *personalistic* as it expresses the personal degree of belief an individual holds that an event will occur. For example, it may be an individual's personal view that a man from a particular population has a DMFT of zero, that a certain person has oral cancer, or that a coin will land on heads when tossed. The subjective view of probability is based on the individual's experiences and his or her ability to amass and construe information from external sources, and may well vary from one individual to another. It can be applied to one-off events.

3. **Model based.** This type of probability, sometimes termed an *a priori* probability, relies on being able to specify all possible equally likely outcomes of an experiment, in advance of or even without carrying out the experiment. So, in the coin tossing example, there are two equally

likely outcomes, a head and a tail. The probability of an event which defines a particular outcome or set of outcomes, if appropriate, is the number of outcomes which relate to the event of interest divided by the total number of outcomes. Thus the probability of a head (the event of interest) is one divided by two (the total number of possible outcomes) which equals $^1/2$. If a card were drawn from a pack of fifty two cards, the *a priori* probability of a 'heart' would be 13 (the number of hearts in the pack) divided by 52 (the number of cards), ie $^1/4$. Clearly, only some situations are amenable to this approach to defining a probability; the probability of a man having a DMFT of zero cannot be assessed in this manner. It is interesting to note that the frequentist probability of an event tends to coincide with, or at least tends towards, the *a priori* probability when the experiment is repeated very many times. Thus, if a fair coin was tossed 10 times, it would not be surprising if 7 heads were obtained (giving a frequentist probability of a head as 0·7), but if the coin were tossed 10,000 times, the proportion of heads would be expected to be very close to 0·5.

Conditional probability

There are various rules that can be adopted to evaluate probabilities of interest. Each will be illustrated by considering drawing a card or two cards from a pack.

1. **Addition rule.** This states that if two events are *mutually exclusive* (this means that if one of the events occurs, the other event cannot occur), then the probability that either one occurs is the sum of the individual probabilities. So for two events, A and B,

$$Pr(A \text{ or } B) = Pr(A) + Pr(B)$$

   Thus the probability of drawing either a heart or a spade from the pack of 52 cards is $^1/4 + ^1/4 = ^1/2 = 0·5$.

2. **Multiplication rule.** This states that if two events are *independent* (this means that the events do not influence each other in any way), then the probability that both of these events occur is equal to the product of the probabilities of each. So,

$$Pr(\text{A and B}) = Pr(\text{A}) \times Pr(\text{B})$$

Thus the probability of drawing the king of hearts is $1/13 \times 1/4 = 1/52 = 0.019$.

If the events are *not independent*, then a different rule, requiring the understanding of a *conditional probability*, has to be adopted. The conditional probability of an event B, written $Pr(\text{B}|\text{A})$ or $Pr(\text{B given A})$, defines the probability of B occurring when it is known that A has already occurred. The rule for dependent events states that the probability of both events occurring is equal to the probability of one times the *conditional* probability of the other. So,

$$Pr(\text{A and B}) = Pr(\text{A}) \times Pr(\text{B given A})$$

For example, suppose that two cards are drawn from the pack and the first is not replaced before the second is taken. The probability of both of these cards being clubs is the product of the probability of the first being a club (ie 13/52) and the second being a club, given that the first was a club (ie 12/51), which is 0·085. Conditional probability plays an important role in Bayesian statistics.

The frequentist philosophy

The most common philosophy underlying statistical analysis is the **frequentist** or **classical** approach, often termed the **Neyman–Pearson** approach, named after the two statisticians who were instrumental in developing the early theory of statistical hypothesis tests. The two features which characterise the frequentist approach are:

1 All the information which is used to make inferences about the attributes of interest in the population is obtained from the sample.

2 The results of the analysis are interpreted in a framework which relates to the long-term behaviour of the experiment in assumed similar circumstances. Thus, the P-value, which is fundamental to the interpretation of the results, is strictly (although it is often misinterpreted) a *frequentist* probability.

Suppose a particular parameter, the population mean, is relevant to an investigation concerned with comparing the effects of a test and a control treatment on a response of interest. A sample of patients is selected and each patient is randomly allocated to one of the two treatments. For example, a double blind randomised trial (Fine et al., 1985)[1] compared the mean wet plaque weight of adults' teeth (collecting the plaque from 20 teeth per adult) when one group of adults received an antiseptic mouthwash and a second group received its vehicle control, each 'treatment' being used twice daily for nine months and in addition to normal tooth brushing. The null hypothesis, H_0, is that the means are the same in the two groups *in the population*. Using the *sample* data, a test statistic is evaluated from which a P-value is determined. The P-value is NOT the probability that the true difference in means is zero. Classicists regard the population attribute (in the above example, the difference in population means) as fixed, so that they cannot attach a probability directly to the attribute. The P-value is the probability of obtaining a difference between sample means equal to or more extreme than that observed, if H_0 is true. That is, if the experiment were to be repeated many times, and H_0 were true, the observed (or a more extreme) difference in means would be obtained on $100P\%$ of occasions. In the same vein, the classicist strictly describes the 95% (say) confidence interval for the true difference in the two means as that interval which, if the experiment were to be repeated on many occasions, would contain the true difference in means on 95% of occasions.

It should be noted that the classical approach to hypothesis testing, because it does not allow a probability to be attached directly to the hypothesis, H_0, dichotomises the results according to whether or not they are 'significant', typically if the P-value is less or greater than 0·05. For this reason, it can be argued that the approach is not well suited to decision making, since the P-value does not give an indication of the extent to which H_0 is false (eg how different the means are). If the sample size is large, the results of a test may be highly significant (ie the P-value very small) even if there is very little difference between the treatment means. Alternatively, the results may be non-significant (ie with a large P-value) if the sample size is small even if there is a large difference between the treatment means.

The Bayesian philosophy

Bayesian statistical methods, developed from the reasoning adopted by an eighteenth century clergyman, the Rev. Thomas Bayes, draw a conclusion about a population parameter by combining information from the sample with initial beliefs about the parameter. More explicitly, the sample data, expressed as a **likelihood** function, is used to modify the **prior** information about the parameter, expressed as a probability distribution and derived from objective and/or subjective sources, to produce what is termed the **posterior** distribution for the parameter.

The Bayesian approach is described in detail in texts such as those by Iversen (1984)[2] and Barnett (1999),[3] and is summarised by Lilford and Braunholtz (1996).[4] It is characterised by the following features which differ quite markedly from those of the classical approach:

1 It incorporates information which is extraneous to the sample data into the calculations. This is the prior information about the parameter of interest.

2 It assumes that the parameter of interest, rather than being fixed, has a probability distribution. Initially, this is the prior distribution but it is updated, using the sample data, to form the posterior distribution. A probability distribution attaches a probability to every possible value of the quantity of interest. This means that, in a Bayesian analysis, it is possible to evaluate the probability that a parameter has a particular value and, consequently, the probability that a null hypothesis about the parameter is true. It is this probability in which most people are interested – the chance that null hypothesis is true – rather than the probability associated with the classical analysis, namely the P-value. Furthermore, a Bayesian can truly interpret a 95% confidence interval as the range of values which contains the true population parameter with 95% certainty, the interpretation often falsely adopted by classicists. The Bayesian point estimate of the parameter is usually taken to be the mode of the posterior distribution, ie its most likely value.

3 It relies on the subjective interpretation of a probability, reflecting a personal degree of belief in an outcome, as the choice of prior depends on the investigator and it is not interpreted in a frequentist manner. This personal belief in a parameter value or the truth of the null hypothesis will probably change as further evidence becomes available. The Bayesian accommodates this reasoning by using the sample data to update the prior into the posterior. Continual updating can be achieved by using this posterior as the prior for the next Bayesian analysis.

The likelihood
Central to the Bayesian philosophy is the likelihood, the probability of getting the data observed in the sample when the parameter of interest takes a particular value (eg the value when H_0 is true). The likelihood for the sample data will be different for different hypotheses about a particular parameter (or parameter specification such as the difference in means), ie for different values of this parameter. It is possible to consider all possible parameter values, and calculate the likelihood in each case, ie the probability of getting the data actually observed in each instance. This can be achieved if the parameter is assumed to follow a known probability distribution, such as the discrete Binomial or the continuous Normal distributions. If these probabilities are plotted against the parameter values, then the resulting plot is called the *likelihood function*.

Bayes theorem
Bayes theorem provides the means of updating the prior probability using sample data, and is the basic tool of Bayesian analysis. Suppose a null hypothesis, H_0, about a particular parameter specification is to be tested, say that the difference in the mean responses between test and control treatments is zero in the population (eg that the difference between the mean plaque weights from adults' teeth after using either a mouthwash or a vehicle control for 9 months is zero). If the prior probability that H_0 is true is $Pr(H_0)$, and the likelihood of getting the data when H_0 is true is $Pr(data|H_0)$, where the vertical line is read as 'given', then Bayes theorem states that the posterior probability that H_0 is true is:

$$Pr(H_0|data) \propto Pr(data|H_0) \, Pr(H_0),$$

ie the posterior probability is proportional to the product of the likelihood and the prior probability. Both the posterior probability and the likelihood are conditional probabilities. Bayes theorem converts the unconditional prior probability into a conditional posterior probability.

In fact, Bayes theorem states that:

$$Pr(H_0|data) = \frac{Pr(data|H_0)Pr(H_0)}{Pr(data)}$$

where the denominator, called the *normalising* constant, is a factor which makes the total probability equal to one when all possible hypotheses are considered. When there are only discrete possibilities for the parameter values, say the set $H_0, H_1, H_2, \ldots, H_k$, then the denominator becomes $\Sigma Pr(\text{data}|H_i)Pr(H_i)$ where the sum extends over all possible values for i, namely $i = 0, 1, 2, \ldots, k$.

When the parameter can take any value within a range of continuous values, then both the prior and posterior probabilities are replaced by probability densities, shown as smooth curves when plotted, with the area under each curve being unity (this corresponds to the sum of all probabilities being one). The posterior density function can then be used to evaluate the probability that the null hypothesis is true (ie that the parameter takes a particular value, say, zero) and also that the parameter takes values within a range such as between one and two.

The choice of prior

One of the factors which has limited the use of Bayesian analysis is the perception that its results are too dependent on an arbitrary factor, namely the choice of prior. In fact, where there is no information from the prior (it is a *non-informative prior* when all possible values for the parameter of interest are equally likely), the prior does not influence the posterior distribution, and the posterior and the likelihood will be proportional. At the other extreme, where the prior provides strong information (for example, when the prior suggests that there is only one possible value for the parameter), the likelihood will not influence the posterior and the posterior will be identical to the prior. Close to these two extremes, there are situations of *vague* and *substantial prior knowledge*. In the former case, the information in the sample data swamps the prior information so that the posterior and likelihood are virtually equal; in the latter case, the posterior departs substantially from the likelihood. To further assuage those in doubt, it is possible to assess how robust conclusions are to changes in the prior distribution by performing a **sensitivity analysis**. Different priors, obtained perhaps from a number of clinicians, lead to a series of posterior distributions. In turn, these may or may not lead to different interpretations of the results, for example, about the extent to which it is believed a novel treatment may be beneficial when compared to an existing therapy.

There are a number of possible types of prior. These include:

1 **Clinical priors** — these express reasonable opinions held by individuals (perhaps clinicians who will participate in the trial) or derived from

published material (such as a meta-analysis of similar studies).

2 **Reference priors** — such priors represent the weakest information (when all possible parameter values are equally likely, ie there is *prior ignorance*), and each is usually used as a baseline against which other priors can be compared.

3 **Sceptical priors** — these priors work on the basis that the effect of interest, such as the treatment effect measured by the difference in treatment means, is close to zero. In such situations, the investigator is sceptical about the effect of treatment, and wants to know the effect on the posterior of the worst plausible outcome.

4 **Enthusiastic priors** — these priors consider the spectrum of opinions which is diametrically opposed to that contained within the community of sceptical priors, namely when the investigator is optimistic about the treatment effect. He or she is interested in the effect on the posterior of the best plausible outcome.

It should be noted that sometimes, when the information extraneous to the sample data is limited, it is difficult or impossible to specify an appropriate prior. Then an **empirical Bayesian analysis**, in which the observed data is used to estimate the prior, may be performed instead of a full Bayesian analysis. Further details may be obtained from Louis (1991).[5]

Applications of the Bayesian method

Although the theory of Bayesian statistics has been around for many years, it has, in the past, been of limited application. This is because, usually, it is very difficult, if not impossible, to calculate the posterior distribution analytically. Instead, simulation techniques, such as Monte Carlo methods, have had to be used to approximate the distributions, and these are extremely computer intensive. However, with the advent of fast, cheap and powerful computers, and specialist software (such as: WinBUGS — www.mrc-bsu.cam.ac.uk/bugs/welcome.shtml), this difficulty has, to a large extent, been overcome, and Bayesian methods are becoming more popular and finding a wider application. Some examples are discussed in the following subsections, more details of which can be obtained in papers such as those by Berry (1993),[6] Spiegelhalter *et al.* (1994),[7] Berry and Stangl (1996),[8] and Fayers *et al.* (1997).[9]

Predictive probabilities

Since the Bayesian approach assumes a probability distribution for a parameter, it is possible to calculate **predictive probabilities** for the parameter values of *future* patients, given the results in the sample. This is impossible in the classical framework which is concerned with calculating the probability of the observed data, given a particular parameter specification. Thus, in the Bayesian framework, the potential exists to use the predictive probability, for example, to decide whether or not a specific future patient will respond to treatment, to predict the required drug dose for an individual, or to decide whether a clinical trial should continue.

Diagnostic and screening tests

One of the easiest applications of the Bayesian approach, and one that was applied early on in the development of the method, is to the problem of diagnosis and screening (covered in Chapter 5, Diagnostic Tests for Oral Conditions). Although a dentist may rely on a formal test to diagnose a particular condition in a patient (oral cancer, say), it would be most unusual if the dentist does not have some preconceived idea of whether or not the patient is diseased. This subjective view might be based on the patient's clinical history and the presence of signs and symptoms (for example, a pre-cancerous lesion such as leucoplakia, erythroplakia, chronic mucocutaneous candidiasis, oral submucous fibrosis, syphilitic glossitis, or sideropenic dysphagia), or, if nothing is known about the patient, it may simply be the prevalence of the condition in the population. It seems sensible to include such information in the diagnosis process, and this can be achieved fairly easily in a Bayesian framework. The preconceived idea is the prior (or pre-test) probability, the result of the diagnostic test (which may be positive or negative) determines the likelihood and Bayes theorem combines the two appropriately to produce the posterior (or post-test) probability that the patient has the condition. Rather than labouring through the mechanical process of applying Bayes theorem, a simple approach is to use Fagan's nomogram (Fig. 1).[10] The posterior probability is found by connecting the pre-test probability to the likelihood ratio, extending the line and noting where it cuts the post-test axis.

Consider the example which was used in Chapter 5 — Diagnostic Tests for Oral Conditions. A 17-month longitudinal study (Kingman *et al.*, 1988)[11] of 541 US adolescents initially aged 10–15 years was conducted with a view to using the child's baseline level of lactobacilli in saliva as a screening test for

Fig. I Fagan's nomogram for interpreting a diagnostic test result. Adapted from Sachett DL, Richardson WS, Rosenberg W, Haynes RB. *Evidence-based Medicine: How to Practice and Teach EBM* (1997) by permission of the publisher Churchill Livingstone

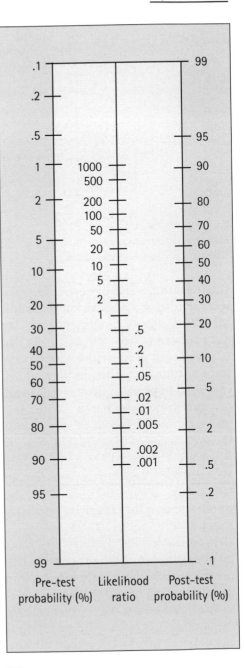

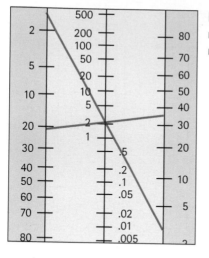

Fig. 2 Two examples of the use of Fagan's nomogram shown by the drawn red lines (a reduced section of Fig. I is shown)

children at high risk of developing caries. A bacterial level of lactobacilli $>10^5$ was regarded as a positive test result and this was compared to the child's caries increment after 17 months, where at least three new lesions in the period were recorded as a positive disease result. Early detection of these high-risk children allows special preventative programmes to be instituted for them, and this is important both for the individual child and for society, as the gain can be expressed in terms of dental health and economy. Suppose that it is of interest to determine whether a particular child from the population under investigation is likely to be at high risk of developing caries. It is known that the prevalence of high risk children (in terms of caries development) in this population is about 21%, and the sensitivity and the specificity of the test are 15% and 93%, respectively. Thus the pre-test probability of the child being high risk can be taken as 0·21 (or 21%), and the likelihood ratio of a positive test result, which is the sensitivity divided by 100 minus the specificity (Petrie and Sabin, 2000),[12] is 15/(100–93) = 2·14. Using Fagan's nomogram and connecting 21% on the left hand axis to 2·14 on the middle axis and extending the line gives a value on the right hand axis of about 35% so that the post-test or posterior probability is approximately equal to 0·35 (Fig. 2). On this basis, it is probably worth investigating the child further (eg by using additional test such as that based on the level of *mutans streptococci* in saliva). If, on the other hand, the child comes from a different population in which the prevalence of high risk children is only 1·5%, then the line connecting 1·5% on the left hand axis to 2·14 on the middle axis cuts the right hand axis at about 3% so that the post-test probability comes to approximately 0·03 (Fig. 2). The pre- and post-test probabilities are both extremely low in this instance, and the child from this population can be regarded as being at very low risk of developing caries, so that no further action needs be adopted for this child. It may be of interest to note that, in each case, the Bayesian post-test or posterior probability determined using Fagan's nomogram corresponds (after allowing for rounding errors and the approximations involved in the use of the nomogram) to the positive predictive value of the test, evaluated in the 'diagnostic tests' chapter.

Clinical trials

The Bayesian approach can be used in clinical trials, both in their design and analysis, when a **decision** has to be made, such as whether or not to admit more patients to a study or to adopt a new therapy. The process requires an assessment of the costs and benefits of the consequences associated with the possible decisions. These consequences are expressed as utilities, and should be specified by an appropriate team of experts (eg dentists, pharmacologists, oncologists etc) who have to address issues relevant to the problem. These utilities are then weighted by the probabilities of the consequences (the predictive probabilities) to determine the expected benefits. The decision that maximises the expected benefit or minimises the maximum loss is then chosen.

Conclusion

The issue of whether or not to adopt a Bayesian approach to statistical analysis in a given circumstance remains controversial and one of personal choice. This paper has attempted to introduce the concepts and highlight the advantages and disadvantages of such procedures. Whatever one's views, however, it should be recognised that the Bayesian approach to data analysis is one of the greatest single developments in statistics since Pearson, Fisher, Gosset (Student) and their colleagues created the theoretical framework of the conventional significance test. After almost a century, and with the advent of powerful computers, the subject 'statistics' may be on the brink of a revolution as important as the change from Newton to Einstein was for Physics. In the early years of the twentieth century there were many sceptics about relativity and atomic physics just as now there are many sceptics among statisticians about the practical usefulness of Bayesian methods. However, the new millennium is still young and even if

Bayesian methods are accepted universally, one wonders if the community of statisticians will be ready for a third revolution after another century!

1 Fine D H, Letizia J, Mandel I D. The effect of rinsing with Listerine antiseptic on the properties of developing dental plaque: *J Clin Periodontol* 1985; 12: 660-666.
2 Iversen G R. *Bayesian statistical inference*. Sage University Paper series on Quantitative Applications in the Social Sciences, series 07-043. Thousand Oaks, California: Sage University Press, 1984.
3 Barnett V. *Comparative statistical inference*. 3rd edn. New York: Wiley, 1999.
4 Lilford R J, Braunholtz D A. The statistical basis of public policy: a paradigm shift is overdue. *Br Med J* 1996; 313: 603-607.
5 Louis T A. Using empirical Bayes methods in biopharmaceutical research. *Stat Med* 1991; 10: 811-829.
6 Berry D A. A case for Bayesianism in clinical trials. *Stat Med* 1993; 12: 1377-1393.
7 Spiegelhalter D J, Freedman L S, Parmar M K B. Bayesian approaches to randomized trials. *J R Statist Soc A* 1994; 157: 357-416.
8 Berry D A, Stangl D K. 'Bayesian methods in health-related research' in *Bayesian Biostatistics*. Eds Berry D A, Stangl D K. New York: Marcel Dekker, 1996.
9 Fayers P M, Ashby D, Parmar M K. Tutorial in biostatistics: Bayesian monitoring in clinical trials. *Stat Med* 1997; 16: 1413-1430.
10 Sachett D L, Richardson N S, Rosenberg W, Haynes R B. *Evidence-based medicine: how to practice adn teach EBM*. London: Churchill Livingstone, 1997.
11 Kingman A, Little W, Gomez I, Heifetz S B, Driscoll W S, Sheats R, Supan P. Salivary levels of Streptococcus mutans and lactobacilli and dental caries experiences in a US adolescent population. *Community Dent Oral Epidemiol* 1988: 16: 98-103.
12 Petrie A, Sabin C. *Medical Statistics at a Glance*. Oxford: Blackwell Science, 2000.

Sherlock Holmes, evidence and evidence-based dentistry

10

If one were to go by the explosion of interest in evidence-based clinical practice in the past decade of the second millennium, one could be forgiven for thinking that the idea was new. In fact, a quick search of *Medline* revealed 9,306 references to 'evidence-based medicine' (EBM) and 291 when the search was restricted to dentistry. It is claimed (Sackett *et al.*, 1996)[1] that the origins of EBM date back to mid-nineteenth century Paris or earlier, although the name EBM was coined in 1992. The inventor of the randomised controlled clinical trial, Sir Austin Bradford Hill, in the 1950s set out the statistical foundations of EBM.

It is not the intention of this chapter to review either the 9,306 articles or the 291 articles or even the substantial contributions made to evidence-based medicine published in the *British Dental Journal*. Rather, the objectives of this chapter are much more general:

1 To describe briefly what is evidence-based medicine and dentistry.

2 To describe the nature of external evidence. To review, very briefly, the philosophy of drawing conclusions from evidence.

3 To describe how evidence can be quantified.

Evidence-based medicine (EBM)

In an important editorial (Sackett *et al.*, 1996) entitled, 'Evidence-Based Medicine: What it is and what it isn't',[1] David Sackett, one of the pioneers of the new movement for the practice of EBM, and his colleagues emphasise that EBM (and by analogy, evidence-based dentistry) has two components '*The practice of EBM means integrating individual clinical expertise with the best available external clinical evidence from systematic research.*' Individual clinical expertise is acquired as a result of clinical practice and means that a clinician is not expected to slavishly follow rules dictated by others when it comes to the treatment of a particular patient. The clinician is likely to know much more about the needs of an individual patient, about the history of the condition, about the social context of the patient including his way of life, his family background, employment situation etc than can be found by reading and learning from research reports, whose main objective is to reach generalised conclusions about 'patients of this type'. As Sherlock Holmes said, *'There is nothing like first hand evidence'*, (Arthur Conan Doyle (ACD): *A Study in Scarlet*, 1888).[2,3] On the other hand, the results of excellent relevant clinical research provide a scientifically valid framework for patient care. According to Sackett *et al.* (1996),[1] *'External clinical evidence both invalidates previously accepted diagnostic tests and treatments and replaces them with new ones that are more powerful, more accurate, more efficacious and safer.'* Or in the words of Holmes, *'The mystery gradually clears away as each new discovery furnishes a step which leads to the complete truth'*, (ACD *The Engineer's Thumb*, 1892). Clearly both components are necessary; clinical expertise without the application of the results of new research is likely to stagnate and cannot be expected to progress without the continuing education provided by good clinical publications. *'Education never ends, Watson. It is a series of lessons with the greatest for the last.'* (ACD *The Adventure of the Red Circle*, 1911).

The nature of external evidence

Evidence is the ultimate product of the analysis of a series of observations. Such a statement may appear banal, but in fact, precise observations are a necessary ingredient for the improvement of clinical expertise and the production of good research. There is a great tendency for all of us to observe what we expect to see rather than what actually occurs. Sometimes this problem can be ameliorated in clinical research by blinding the patient and the clinical observer and yes, even the statistician. Sir Arthur Conan Doyle was a medical practitioner and it is said that he modelled his fictional detective, Sherlock Holmes, on one of his professors at Edinburgh Medical School, Dr Joseph Bell (1837–1911). Bell was thought by his students to be a magician. In Doyle's words, *'Dr Bell would sit in a receiving room, with a face like a Red Indian, and diagnose people as they came in, before they even opened their mouths. He would tell them their symptoms and even give them details of their past life and hardly ever would make a mistake'.*

Although the philosophical origins of EBM date back to the mid-nineteenth century, its legal status in Britain was implied by the Apothecaries Act of 1815, which licensed apothecaries in order to protect the public from the growing number of unqualified druggists and herbalists. The Medical Act of 1858 led to the creation of the medical register which contained the names of all doctors with recognised medical qualifications. The 1858 Act restricted the practice of medicine to those doctors included in the register. There was also the implication that these doctors should practice 'real' medicine, that is, the medicine taught and learned in medical schools, and the public would be protected against charlatans. The Act was not successful in eliminating complementary or alternative medicine, and indeed, apart from a short period in the middle of the twentieth century, the number of people who seek medical help outside the official medical profession, particularly from herbalists, has continued to increase. (Paradoxically, alternative medicine is still promoted and supplied by chemist's shops, the very place where a patient, having consulted a regular doctor, is required to go to collect his prescription! Boots, the chemists, even publish and distribute free a booklet (Anon, 2000)[4] in which complementary medicine is stated to be safe, and it is implied that orthodox medical help need be sought only where symptoms are severe and persistent). The 1858 Act implied that the medicine practised by registered doctors was based on evidence while the alternative was based on hearsay, old-wives-tales, grannies' remedies etc. If this distinction was one of the objectives of the 1858 Act, it most certainly was not very successful; there are many examples, in all medical specialities, of practice which, either for lack of evidence or ignorance, is not based on evidence. For example, Mills et al. (1994) showed that a much publicised and widely sold pre-brushing mouthwash was ineffective in reducing plaque or stains in comparison with a control,[5] while Scherer et al. (1998) showed that a herbal mouth rinse significantly reduced gingival bleeding.[6] Some controversies seem never to be resolved because of the difficulty of obtaining sufficient clear-cut evidence one way or the other. Is the use of mercury amalgams totally without risk? Even if the dental profession is convinced of its safety, there are many that would not seem to be. Should pathology free impacted third molars be extracted prophylactically? Bandolier[7] answers by asking, 'What do you do when there is no evidence? Carry on with what you are doing because you have no evidence to stop, or stop what you are doing because there is no evidence to carry on?'. Similarly, Alexander (1998) has identified eleven myths of dentoalveolar surgery, and so on.[8]

The weight of the evidence derived from a clinical study will depend on its design and how well it has been conducted. A simple case series reporting a new treatment may not provide very strong evidence of the effect of the treatment unless the observed effect is exceedingly different from the natural progress of the disease or condition. On the other hand, a case series may be sufficient to generate a hypothesis which might be investigated by more rigorous studies. A control group will always increase the validity of a study based on a case series.

As noted in Chapter 3, Clinical Trials I, randomisation of the patients to the treatment groups will tend to remove the effect of confounding factors especially if the trial is not too small. Thus in terms of a single study, the randomised controlled trial (RCT) provides the best evidence that a treatment has an effect in comparison with the control group. This evidence is usually presented in the form of a significance test and a confidence interval for the treatment effect.

When there are several studies of the effect of a particular treatment, the results may be aggregated using the techniques of meta-analysis (Chapter 8), another new name for an old idea. '*There is nothing new under the sun, it has all been done before.*' (ACD. *A Study in Scarlet*,1888). To learn of the pitfalls of combining evidence in a meta-analysis, there is no better starting point than the early article by Daniels and Bradford Hill (1952).[9] A good meta-analysis should take account of the study designs, involve a well defined strategy for literature searches, assessment of quality, inclusion and exclusion criteria, tests of homogeneity etc, although in 1991, Thompson and Pocock (1991) felt that it was necessary to pose the question: can meta-analysis be trusted?[10] In the true spirit of meta-analysis, Holmes pleads, '*Any truth is better than infinite doubt*' (ACD. *The Yellow Face*, 1893).

A review should bring together all the evidence for and against the effectiveness of a treatment, and there may be no simple clear-cut result. Further, there may be more than one review, and what should be done if the reviews differ in their conclusions? On the question of the extraction of impacted third molars, Bandolier suggests that the quality of the reviews be judged, and if they do not contain randomised controlled trials, they should be regarded with '*a cold and fishy eye*', which leaves us just about where we started by asking the question: what should the clinician do, stop or carry on? However, for a given patient, the clinician must make a decision and may not have the luxury Holmes enjoyed when he said in honesty to Watson, '*No, no; I never guess. It is a shocking habit – destructive to the logical faculty*' (ACD. *The Sign of the Four*, 1890).

If the reviews do agree, a review of the reviews may evolve into a clinical guideline. One might be forgiven for thinking that at this point there would no longer be controversy, but not so. Whether created locally or nationally or internationally, guidelines are generally an aggregation of research evidence, expert opinion and clinical experience. The existence of a clinical guideline may intentionally have the effect of limiting the freedom of action of a clinician in the treatment of his patient, and this could have legal consequences and ethical implications. Holmes is mistaken when he says of Dr Grimesby Roylott *'When a doctor does go wrong, he is the first of criminals. He has nerve and the knowledge.'* (ACD: *The Speckled Band* 1892). Holmes is speaking of going wrong in a legal sense rather than making a mistaken clinical judgement, but unfortunately a clinician rarely has all the knowledge, and errors will occur. Hurwitz (1998) expounds a comprehensive and highly readable account of the possible legal implications of following or not following clinical guidelines in his book appropriately titled *Clinical Guidelines and the Law; Negligence, Discretion and Judgement.*[11] These implications are important because the existence of guidelines neither implies that they will be followed in practice nor that their effectiveness will be formally evaluated. Not surprisingly, after meta-analyses of meta-analyses and reviews of reviews, there is also a *Guide to Guidelines* (Smith, 1997)![12]

Evidence and the philosophy of scientific progress

The above title of this chapter is nothing but presumptuous when one thinks of the miles of shelves of books and other publications on this subject produced over the past 100 years, but statistics has played an important, under-rated and often overlooked role in the theories propounded by professional philosophers. Healy (2000) has recently published an entertaining but serious discussion of the role of statistics in the philosophy of science, and the philosophy of science in the practice of statistics.[13] In essence, the modern subject, 'statistics', has its origins at University College London around the start of the twentieth century when Karl Pearson began studying the theory of distributions and applying statistical methods to study biological problems, and, for example, discovered the chi-squared distribution and began thinking in terms of the significance test. Pearson's ideas were expanded and developed in the 1920s and 1930s by Fisher, and Gossett (the ever famous 'student' who first described the *t*-test)[14] perfected the idea of the statistical significance test which has remained with us, virtually without change, until today. Basically the logical procedure followed in a statistical significance test is:

1 A stimulus provokes the need to perform an experiment to compare the effects of say, two treatments, A and B, on an outcome. The origin and form of the stimulus is not important and may come from a clinical observation, a hunch, hearsay, complimentary medicine etc. If the stimulus is based on evidence, this evidence cannot be used further in the experiment, and the experiment to compare the two treatments will be interpreted with a completely open mind, ignoring all that is known before (unless a Bayesian approach, discussed in chapter 9, is used).

2 A null hypothesis is formulated, which states that the treatment effect (eg that the average difference between the two treatments) is zero. This hypothesis represents the state of knowledge at the start of the experiment and relates to the population of values.

3 The results of the experiment, derived from sample data, are analysed to discover if they provide sufficient evidence to reject the null hypothesis and thus change the state of knowledge by concluding that one treatment is better than the other. *'It is a capital mistake to theorise before one has the data. Insensibly one begins to twist the facts to suit the theories, instead of the theories to suit the facts'.* (ACD. *A Scandal in Bohemia*, 1892). The decision to reject the null hypothesis, however, is based on probabilistic reasoning. Actually, it is the frequency or repeated experiment approach to probability as opposed to subjective probability or *a priori* probability reasoning. A single patient cannot of him or herself disprove the null hypothesis. *'We balance probabilities and choose the most likely. It is the scientific use of the imagination.'* (ACD. *The Hound of the Baskervilles*, 1901-2).

4 A confidence interval for the effect of interest, such as the average difference between the treatments, is constructed. This should enable the researcher to determine whether or not there is sufficient evidence to conclude that the difference between the treatments is of *clinical* importance.

In fact, it was some decades later that the most influential philosopher of science of the twentieth century, Sir Karl Popper (1959 and 1972),[15,16] re-proposed that science advances, a step at a time, by the refutation of hypotheses. It seems that the statisticians were expert Popperians long before Popper's theories became popular. Fisher (1937), anticipating Popper by almost twenty years, stated *'Every experiment may be said to exist only in order to give the facts a chance of disproving the null hypothesis.'* and this assertion was based on a complex form of probabilistic reasoning.[14]

Later, Popper's theory was challenged by Thomas Kuhn (1966), who argued that while science generally progresses slowly and steadily, there were events of dramatic importance, or revolutions, which totally changed the state of knowledge.[17] One can easily think of examples of such revolutions which have transformed scientific thinking: the introduction into Europe of the decimal number system by Leonardo di Pisa (Fibonacci) in 1202, enabling complex arithmetic to be performed and providing the trigger for the start of the renaissance, Galileo, Newton, Einstein's theory of relativity etc. However, revolutions also occur within specialities and in dentistry one can think of examples, such as the discovery of effective anaesthetics, the invention of the first high speed flexible shaft dental drill by Samuel Stockton White in 1844, the adoption of mercury based amalgams for fillings instead of gold about 160 years ago, or the discovery of the role of fluoride in the prevention of childhood caries. The introduction of randomisation in clinical trials by Bradford Hill was a revolution in medical statistics,[18] and it seems that maybe we are experiencing now a Kuhnian revolution in the form of the Bayesian approach to evidence from clinical studies. If indeed the subject, 'statistics', is transformed totally by the adoption of Bayesian techniques, it will be necessary to re-think what is meant by evidence based on Popperian inference in relation to medical practice. However, for the near or medium future, the validity and strength of evidence will continue to be based on Fisher-Popper statistical significance tests and their associated confidence intervals. Perhaps sadly, we are likely to witness for many more years the spectacle of our normally calm, serious, reserved research worker, suddenly triumphant and exuberant as his computer prints out the long awaited and much desired $P < 0.05$.

Presenting statistical evidence

We all know that there is not much difference between a half-full glass and one that is half-empty, but the results of even the simplest research can be presented in a bewildering variety of ways. Consider the simplest clinical trial in which a new treatment is to be compared with the existing standard treatment and the

Table I 2x2 table of frequencies

	New treatment	Standard treatment	Total	
Success	a	b	$a+b$	total number of successes
Failure	c	d	$c+d$	total number of failures
Total	n_1	n_2	n	total number of patients

outcome is dichotomous, a success or a failure. The results would usually be set out in the form of Table 1, a two by two table of frequencies. The number of ways of comparing the two treatments and their associated tests of significance and confidence intervals seem limitless.

Comparison by the difference between the two success rates

Suppose the proportions of patients whose treatment result in a success are $p_1=a/n_1$ for the new and $p_2=b/n_2$ for the standard treatment. (These sample proportions are often referred to as the estimated success rates even if they are not strictly rates; in the population, the true success 'rates' are π_1 and π_2). The null hypothesis is that the two treatments have an equal chance of success (ie $\pi_1 = \pi_2$). The statistical significance of the difference between p_1 and p_2 can be determined by calculating $z_1 = (p_1 - p_2)/\text{SE}(p_1 - p_2)$ which follows the standardized Normal distribution, or equivalently, by calculating z_1^2 which follows the chi-squared distribution with one degree of freedom [*note*: $\text{SE}(p_1 - p_2)$ is the standard error of $(p_1 - p_2)$]. A continuity correction should be applied to z_1 and to the chi-squared test statistic but it has relatively little effect if the sample sizes are not too small. The 95% confidence interval for the true difference in the two success rates is $(p_1 - p_2) \pm 1.96\text{SE}(p_1 - p_2)$. These expressions for the significance test and the confidence interval assume that the values of a, b, c and d are not too small but if that were the case, Fisher's exact significance test would be an appropriate alternative to z_1 or the chi-squared test statistic.

Comparison by the difference between the two failure rates

This is the half-empty version of the half-full glass. If the observed proportion of patients whose treatment fails is q_1 for the new and q_2 for the standard treatment, the difference between them is the same as the difference between the two success rates. Thus the significance of the difference between the two failure rates and the confidence interval for the difference are identical to those of the difference in success rates.

Comparison by the ratio of the two success rates

If the ratio of the two success rates is $R_1 = p_1/p_2$, the sampling distribution of R_1 is log-Normal. Then the hypothesis that the ratio of the true success rates is one can be tested by calculating $z_2 = \log_e R_1/SE(\log_e R_1) = \log_e R_1/\sqrt{(q_1/a + q_2/b)}$ which follows the standardized Normal distribution. It should be noted that z_2 is not exactly equal to z_1. The 95% confidence interval for the ratio of the true success rates is obtained by calculating the exponential of the two limits for $\log_e$ of this ratio, ie the exponential of $\log_e R_1 \pm 1 \cdot 96 SE(\log_e R_1)$.

Comparison by the ratio of the two failure rates

If the ratio of the two failure rates is $R_2 = q_2/q_1$, the Standard Normal Deviate for testing the significance of the ratio of the true failure rates is $z_3 = \log_e R_2/SE(\log_e R_2) = \log_e R_2/\sqrt{(p_1/c + p_2/d)}$ which is not exactly equal to z_1 or z_2. The 95% confidence interval for the ratio of the true failure rates is obtained by calculating the exponential of the two limits for $\log_e$ of this ratio, ie the exponential of $\log_e R_2 \pm 1 \cdot 96 SE(\log_e R_2)$.

Comparison by the odds ratio of success and the odds ratio of failure

The observed odds of a success for the new treatment is a/c and for the standard treatment it is b/d. The observed odds ratio for a success is thus $OR_1 = (a/c)/(b/d) = (ad)/(bc)$; the Standard Normal Deviate for testing the significance of the true odds ratio for a success is:

$$z_4 = \log_e OR_1/SE(\log_e OR_1)$$
$$= \log_e OR_1/\sqrt{(1/a + 1/b + 1/c + 1/d)}$$

A 95% confidence interval for the true odds ratio is the exponential of the limits for $\log_e$ of this ratio, ie the exponential of

$$\log_e OR_1 \pm 1 \cdot 96\sqrt{(1/a + 1/b + 1/c + 1/d)}$$

The value of z_4 is not exactly equal to z_1, z_2 or z_3. If instead of the odds of a success, the odds of failure are considered, $OR_2 = (bc)/(ad)$ which is the

Table 2 Results of the analyses of three examples of hypothetical trials								
		Example 1		Example 2		Example 3		
Observed frequencies								
	new	standard	new	standard	new	standard	new	standard
Success	a	b	10	5	20	10	80	40
Failure	c	d	90	95	80	90	20	60
Estimated effects								
diff. p_1-p_2			0·10-0·05=0·05		0·20-0·10=0·10		0·80-0·40=0·40	
diff. q_2-q_1			0·95-0·90=0·05		0·90-0·80=0·10		0·60-0·20=0·40	
ratio p_1/p_2			2·000		2·000		2·000	
ratio q_2/q_1			1·056		1·125		3·000	
OR for success (new/standard)			2·111		2·250		6·000	
Test statistics								
z_1 (difference)			1·34		1·98		5·77	
z_1 (corrected)			1·23		1·78		5·63	
z_2 (ratio p_1/p_2)			1·31		1·92		5·24	
z_3 (ratio q_2/q_1)			1·34		1·96		5·09	
z_4 (odds ratio)			1·32		1·95		5·55	
P-values								
P_1 (difference)			0·180		0·048		<0·000001	
P_1 (corrected)			0·283		0·075		<0·000001	
P_1 (Fisher exact)			0·283		0·073		<0·000001	
P_2 (ratio p_1/p_2)			0·190		0·055		<0·000001	
P_3 (ratio q_2/q_1)			0·182		0·050		<0·000001	
P_4 (odds ratio)			0·188		0·051		<0·000001	

reciprocal of OR_1. The Standard Normal Deviate for the test of significance of the true odds ratio of a failure is $-z_4$ and the 95% confidence interval is the reciprocal of that for the odds ratio of a success. The odds ratio gives equivalent results from the significance tests for both success and failure.

Comparison of the different methods

These four methods are probably the most commonly used of the very many methods of summarising a 2×2 table of frequencies. Table 2 shows the bewildering array of results obtained from applying these methods to three simple examples. In each of the three examples the new treatment doubles the success rate of the old treatment. However, it can be seen that the method of comparison may give different impressions of the improvement offered by the new treatment even if the methods only produce slightly different Standard Normal Deviates for the significance test of the null hypothesis, and slightly different P-values.

In the first example, the success rates for the standard and the new treatments are both low (ie 0·05 and 0·10) and hence the difference between them is small. The new treatment doubles the success rate but the old method only increases the failure rate by 5·6% (ie 5/90 × 100%)! The Fisher exact test and the corrected Standard Normal Deviate (or, equivalently, the corrected chi-squared test) give the same P-values, which are different from those obtained using the other methods. This is because the 2×2 table contains small frequencies (the numbers of patients with a successful outcome are 5 and 10) and the corrected and Fisher exact values are probably the most reliable, the other P-values being too small because of the lack of the continuity correction.

The second example is even more perplexing. The ratio of the two success rates is two and the odds ratio is 2·25 but using the old treatment only increases the risk of failure by 12·5%! If a decision were to be made on the basis of the 5% level of significance there would be even greater difficulty, since for some comparisons $P \leq 0.05$ while for others $P > 0.05$! Again in this example, the Fisher test and the corrected Standard Normal Deviate are probably the most reliable and the conclusion should be that the difference is not statistically significant at the 5% level.

In the third example, the success rates are comparatively large and there are no very low frequencies in the 2×2 table. The new treatment doubles the chance of success from 40% to 80% and increases the odds of success 6-fold whilst the use of the old treatment triples the risk of failure. The values of z, although slightly different, lead to exactly the same interpretation, that it is most unlikely that the observed difference between the treatments is due merely to chance.

The discussion of these three examples has concentrated on statistical significance only because the evaluation of evidence is to a large degree based on the Fisher–Popperian philosophy that only by the refutation of hypotheses can scientific knowledge progress. It is left as an exercise for the reader to calculate the associated confidence intervals, which would be essential if the usefulness of a real new treatment were to be evaluated in comparison with the old. Although the data in the three examples are hypothetical, it may be disturbing that even with objective statistical analysis, the results may be open to different interpretations. It is not just a case of a glass being half full or half empty. As Holmes observed '*There is nothing more deceptive than an obvious fact*' (ACD *The Boscombe Valley Mystery*, 1891).

The number needed to treat (NNT)

Because it can be difficult to interpret differences between treatments, other methods of comparing treatments that have a more direct clinical interpretation have been investigated. One of these, the '*number needed to treat*' (NNT) is becoming increasingly popular. McQuay and Moore (1997) give a full description of the method,[19] but the basic idea is to calculate the number of patients that need to have the new treatment instead of the old in order to have one additional patient benefit or, equivalently, prevent one adverse outcome. In the third of the examples discussed earlier, the success rates are 0·80 and 0·40 in the new and standard treatment groups, respectively. The 2x2 table shows that if 100 patients have the new treatment instead of the old, there will be 40 more successes. Thus to achieve just one more success, it will be necessary to give 100/40 =2·5 patients the new treatment. It is not difficult to see that the NNT is just the reciprocal of the difference between the two success rates.

Thus NNT $= 1/(p_1-p_2) = 1/(0·8 - 0·4) = 1/0·40 = 2·5$, or equivalently NNT $= 1/(q_2-q_1)$.

Since the standard error of (p_1-p_2) in this example is:

$$\sqrt{[p_1(1-p_1)/n_1 + p_2(1-p_2)/n_2]} = 0·0632,$$

the 95% confidence interval for the true difference is $0·40 \pm 1·96 \times 0·0632$, or 0·276 to 0·524. Thus the 95% confidence interval for the true NNT is 1·9 to 3·6 (ie 1/0·524 to 1/0·276). The values of NNT to achieve one more success for the first and second examples are 20 and 10 patients, respectively.

The possible values for NNT range from one, when the old treatment is useless and the new is perfect, to infinity when there is no difference between the treatments. Not only does it express the result of the comparison between the treatments in terms of a number of patients, and thus a concept more readily grasped by a clinician than, for example, an odds ratio, but also it may have direct application in the cost/benefit analysis of the decision to adopt the new treatment. This is not to say that the other measures are never useful: indeed each one may be appropriate for a given situation. In an example from dentistry, discussed in Chapter 8, a review (Rijkom *et al.*, 1997) of the usefulness of fluoride gel for the prevention of caries, showed that the overall effect of the gel is to reduce the incidence of caries by 22% per year.[20] Calculations showed that, if without the gel the incidence of caries were 0·25 DMFS per year, it would be necessary to treat 18 teeth with the gel for a year in order to save one DMFS. The NNT decreased to 9, 4·5 and 3 if the incidences without the gel were 0·50, 1·00 and 1·50 DMFS per year, respectively. This example is particularly interesting because it demonstrates that where caries is more prevalent, the NNT is less; in other words, where caries is rare, it may not be worthwhile to use the gel, but where it is common, it might be very cost effective indeed.

Some guidelines

So, recognising the many problems facing the clinician, how can he/she use the evidence-based approach to greatest effect? According to the guidelines propounded by Sackett *et al.* (2000), the following sequence of steps, incorporating the statisical principles described in earlier chapters, should be pursued:[21]

Step 1 Convert the need for information about prevention, diagnosis, prognosis, therapy, etc, into an an answerable question which relates specifically to the patient's requirements and the population of interest.

Step 2 Track down the best evidence with which to answer that question using, for example, MEDLINE and evidence databases (such as Evidence-based Medicine Reviews from Ovid Technologies (www.ovid.com) which combines several electronic databases including the Cochrane Database of Systematic Reviews).

Step 3 Critically appraise the evidence for its validity (closeness to the truth), impact (size of the effect), and applicability (usefulness in clinical practice). This involves ensuring that sources of potential bias have been eliminated, that the appropriate statistical methods have been used, and that all the important outcomes have been considered and are appropriately summarised (eg rates, NNT) with confidence intervals so that a decision can be made as to whether or not the results are clinically important.

Step 4 Integrate the critical appraisal with clinical expertise and with the patient's unique biology, values and circumstances.

Step 5 Finally, evaluate performance in terms of effectiveness and efficiency by questioning the ability to complete steps 1–4 successfully, and seek ways to improve performance in the future.

Conclusion

It is well known that the number of research journals and research papers increases at an alarming rate every year. It would be hoped that the growth in the number of good research reports is equally rapid. If this is in fact the case, in future it will be ever more difficult to identify good research and maintain a register of valid evidence. The Cochrane Foundation, the National Health Service Centre for Reviews and Dissemination at the University of York and others have taken an enormous step forward by trying to filter out the valid evidence from the bulk of less worthy research. Certainly individual clinicians cannot be expected to read all the latest research reports in their field, let alone evaluate them and classify the results as good evidence or not. *I consider that a man's brain is like a little empty attic, and you have to stock it with such furniture as you choose. A fool takes in all the lumber of every sort that he comes across, so that the knowledge which might be useful to him gets crowded out, or at best is jumbled up with a lot of other things, so that he has a difficulty in laying his hands upon it. Now the skilful workman is very careful indeed as to what he takes into his brain-attic. He will have nothing but the tools which may help him in doing his work, but of these he has a large assortment, and all in the most perfect order. It is a mistake to think that that little room has elastic walls and can distend to any extent. Depend upon it — there comes a time when for every addition of knowledge you forget something you knew before. It is of the highest importance, therefore, not to have useless facts elbowing out the useful ones.* (ACD *A Study in Scarlet*, 1887). A clinician, therefore, either must become ever more specialised and remember only the very important aspects of his narrow field, or he can remain a general practitioner but he has to accept that in many situations he will have to consult his 'library'. Nowadays, it is almost essential to have a computer to keep the lumber-room in an accessible order and enable easy contact to be made with such organisations as the Cochrane Foundation and the NHS Centre for Reviews and Dissemination.

Sir Arthur Conan Doyle and his mentor, Dr Joseph Bell, were acutely aware of the value of good evidence in medical practice and for the detective work of Sherlock Holmes. The 60 stories involving Holmes and his assistant Dr Watson were published between 1887 and 1927 in the *Strand Magazine, Colliers Weekly* and other periodicals. They have given pleasure to generations of avid readers eager to discover something of the extraordinary ability of Sherlock Holmes to deduce the truth from whatever evidence was available. Pearson, Fisher,

126

'Student', Popper and others have formalised the idea of the use of evidence to test hypotheses and enable science to progress. Bell, Sackett, his colleagues and others have sought to identify from the mass of available research evidence what is valid and can be realistically applied in the every day practice of clinical medicine.

1 Sackett D L, Rosenberg W M C, Gray J A M, Haynes R B, Richardson W S. Evidence-based medicine: what it is and what it isn't. *Br Med J* 1996 ; 3 1 2: 71-72.
2 All the Sherlock Holmes stories may be found in *Arthur Conan Doyle* (1981) or at www.sherlockian.net/canon/index.html
3 Arthur Conan Doyle (1981) *The Penguin Complete Sherlock Holmes*. Penguin
4 Anon (2000) Your guide to choosing holistic medicines. *Complementary Medicine* The Boots Company PLC, Nottingham, England.
5 Mills D C, Smith S R, Chung L. The effect of using a pre-brushing mouthwash (Plax) on removal of tooth stain in vivo and in vitro. *J Clin Periodont* 1994; 2 1: 13-16.
6 Scherer W, Gultz J, Sangwoo Lee S, Kaim J. The ability of a herbal mouthrinse to reduce gingival bleeding. *J Clin Dent* 1998; 9: 97-100.
7 Bandolier. Prophylactic removal of impacted third molars. http://www.jr2.ox.ac.uk/Bandolier/band42/b42-2.html
8 Alexander R E. Eleven myths of dentoaveolar surgery. *J Am Dent Assoc* 1998; 1 29: 1271-1279.
9 Daniels M, Hill A B. Chemotherapy of pulmonary tuberculosis in young adults; an analysis of the combined results of three Medical Research Council Trials. *Br Med J* 1952; i:1 162-1168.
10 Thompson S G, Pocock S. Can meta-analysis be trusted? *Lancet* 1991; 3 3 8: 1127-1130.
11 Hurwitz B. *Clinical Guidelines and the Law, Negligence, Discretion and Judgement.* Radcliffe Medical Press, Abingdon, 1998.
12 Smith P. (ed) *Guide to the Guidelines: Disease management made simple.* Abingdon: Radcliffe Medical Press, 1997.
13 Healy M J R. *Paradigms and Pragmatism: Approaches to Medical Statistics.* Ann Ig 2000; 12.
14 Fisher R A. Prof Karl Pearson and the method of moments. *Ann Eugenics* 1937; 7: 303-318.
15 Popper K. *Conjectures and Refutations.* 4th ed., London: Routeledge and Kegan Paul, 1972.
16 Popper K. *The Logic of Scientific Discovery.* London: Hutchinson, 1959.
17 Kuhn T. *The structure of Scientific revolutions.* 3rd ed. The University of Chicago Press, 1966.
18 Medical Research Council. Streptomycin treatment of pulmonary tuberculosis. *Br Med J* 1948; 769-782.
19 McQuay H J, Moore R A. Using numerical results from systematic reviews in clinical practice. *Ann Int Med* 1997; 1 26: 712-720.
20 Van Rijkom H M, Truin G J, Van't Hof M A. A meta-analysis of clinical studies on the caries-inhibiting effect of fluoride gel treatment. *Caries Res* 1998; 3 2: 83-92.
21 Sackett D L, Strauss S E, Richardson W S, Rosenberg W, Haynes R B. *Evidence-based Medicine: How to Practice and Teach EBM.* 2nd Edn. Churchill Livingstone, 2000.

Glossary

$\pm$	This means that the quantity following the sign is first subtracted from and then added to the quantity preceding it. Hence, $x \pm y$ is the same as $(x - y)$ and $(x + y)$.
$\propto$	This means that the quantity before the sign is proportional to the quantity after the sign
$\sqrt{}$	The square root
$\geq$	The quantity before the sign is greater than or equal to the quantity after it
$>$	The quantity before the sign is greater than the quantity after it.
$\leq$	The quantity before the sign is less than or equal to the quantity after it.
$<$	The quantity before the sign is less than the quantity after it.
α	The Greek letter 'alpha'. It may refer to the constant term in a regression equation (which is estimated in the sample by a). Alternatively, it sometimes refers to the probability of making a Type I error (rejecting the null hypothesis when it is true) in hypothesis testing.
β	The Greek letter 'beta' which usually refers to the true value of a regression coefficient in a regression model (it is estimated by b in the sample). In simple regression in which there is only one explanatory variable, it represents the slope or gradient of the line. It is also sometimes used to refer to the probability of making a Type II error (not rejecting the null hypothesis when it is false) in hypothesis testing.
$1 - \beta$	In the situation in which β represents the probability of making a Type II error, $1-\beta$ is the power of a hypothesis test. The power is the probability of rejecting the null hypothesis when it is false, ie correctly concluding that there is a treatment effect. Power is often expressed in percentage terms.
β_i	The true partial regression coefficient in a multiple or logistic

regression model (it is estimated in the sample by β_i).

χ The Greek letter 'chi' used to denote a particular probability distribution with known and tabulated percentage points enabling the P-value relating to the chi-squared test of proportions to be evaluated from it.

δ The Greek letter 'delta' which is sometimes used to refer to a clinically or biologically important difference of interest in the population; this usually needs to be specified in sample size calculations.

μ The Greek letter 'mu' which represents the population mean (if the variable of interest is x, this mean is estimated in the sample by $\bar{x}$). It is equal to the sum of all the observations divided by the number of observations on that variable in the population.

π The Greek letter 'pi' which represents the proportion of individuals in the population possessing some characteristic (it is estimated by p in the sample).

θ The Greek letter 'theta' which may be used to represent the overall population effect of treatment in a meta-analysis (it is estimated in the sample by $\hat{\theta}$).

$\hat{\theta}$ The estimated overall effect of treatment obtained from a meta-analysis based on sample data (it estimates the overall population effect, θ)

θ_i The estimated effect of treatment in the ith study in a meta-analysis.

ρ The Greek letter 'rho' which represents the population value of the Pearson product-moment correlation coefficient (it is estimated in the sample by r).

σ The Greek letter 'sigma' which represents the population standard deviation which is a measure of spread of the observations (its estimate obtained from the sample is usually denoted by s).

σ^2 The population variance, ie the square of the standard deviation.

Σ The Greek capital letter 'sigma' which represents the summation sign (see $\sum_{i=1}^{n} x_i$)

2×2 table This is a table which has two rows and two columns and in which the entries are frequencies.

a The constant term in an estimated regression model (it estimates the population value, α). In simple linear regression in which there is only one explanatory variable, it represents the estimated intercept of the line.

ANOVA The analysis of variance.

AUC Area under the curve.

b Often used to refer to an estimated regression coefficient in a regression model (it estimates the population regression coefficient, β).

CI Confidence interval. Strictly, the 95% CI will contain the true parameter on 95% of occasions on repeated sampling; it is usually interpreted (this is the Bayesian interpretation) to mean that there is a 95% chance that the CI contains the parameter of interest.

D– An individual without the disease

D+ An individual with the disease

df The degrees of freedom of a statistic

DMFS The number of decayed, missing or filled surfaces

e This is the exponential, ie a constant equal to $2 \cdot 71828$

e^x This is the exponential function, sometimes written $\exp(x)$. If $x = \log_e(y)$, then $y = e^x$ is the antilogarithm of $\log_e(y)$. Thus, if the logarithmic transformation has been taken of a variable, it can be transformed back to its original scale by taking the antilog, (perhaps using the exponential function of a calculator).

F A particular continuous probability distribution with known and tabulated percentage points so that the P-value relating to the F-test can be evaluated from it. The test statistic for the F-test is often denoted by F.

F-test A hypothesis test which compares two population variances by determining the ratio of the relevant sample variances. In the analysis of variance, the F-test is also used to compare two or more means.

H_0 The null hypothesis (pronounced H nought) that is under investigation in a hypothesis test. It is the hypothesis of no effect in the population (eg no difference in the means in the population).

log x This is the logarithm (log) of the quantity 'x' (ie log x). Sometimes brackets are put around the x to aid clarification (ie log(x)). Logarithms can have different bases, the most usual being 10 (written $\log_{10}$) and e (written $\log_e$ or ln). Note that the log of zero is infinity, and logs cannot be taken of negative numbers. If there are two numbers, a and b, say, then

    (i)   log(a multiplied by b) = log(a) + log(b)

    (ii) log(a divided by b) = log(a) − log(b).

$\log_e x$ This is the Naperian or natural logarithm of x to base e, often written as ln x, where e is the constant 2·71828. If $\log_e(x) = z$ then the antilogarithm of $\log_e(x)$ is $x = e^z$. These natural logs are used more often in statistics than logs with other bases, and are generally used in computer packages.

Logit(p) This is the logistic or logit transformation of the proportion, p, where $\text{logit}(p) = \log_e \dfrac{p}{1-p}$.

n The number of individuals in the sample.

N The number of individuals in the population.

NNT The number needed to treat, ie the number of patients needed to be treated with the new treatment instead of the old treatment in order to prevent one adverse outcome or achieve one more success

NPV The negative predictive value of a diagnostic or screening test. It is the proportion of those testing negative who really are disease-free

OHQoL Oral health quality of life

OR The odds ratio. This is the odds of success in one group of

p individuals (eg those receiving treatment) divided by the odds of success in another group (eg those receiving placebo)

p The proportion of 'successes' in a sample, i.e., the proportion of individuals in the sample possessing some characteristic (it estimates the true population proportion, π). So if there are n individuals in the sample, and r of them possess the characteristic, then $p = r/n$. A proportion can take a value equal to or between zero and one; it can be transformed into a percentage by multiplying it by 100.

$\bar{p}$ The arithmetic mean of two or more sample proportions.

P The P-value obtained in a hypothesis test. It is the probability of obtaining the observed results (or more extreme results) if the null hypothesis is true.

P_i The proportion of individuals possessing some characteristic in the ith group of the sample.

PPV   The positive predictive value of a diagnostic or screening test. It is the proportion of those testing positive who actually have the disease.

$Pr(A|B)$ The conditional probability that event A will occur given that event B has occurred.

$Pr(A)$ The probability that the event 'A' will occur. A probability is equal to or lies between zero and one. A probability can be expressed in percentage terms by multiplying it by 100.

r The sample estimate of the Pearson product-moment correlation coefficient which provides a measure of linear association between two variables, x and y (it estimates the population correlation coefficient, ρ).

$$r = \frac{\Sigma(x-\bar{x})(y-\bar{y})}{\sqrt{\Sigma(x-\bar{x})^2\Sigma(y-\bar{y})^2}}$$

r^2 The proportion of variance in one variable explained by its linear relationship with another variable. It is the square of the correlation coefficient.

R^2 The coefficient of determination. It is the proportion of the variance of the response variable, y, explained by its relationship with the explanatory variables in a multiple regression analysis.

ROC   Receiver operating characteristic.

RCT   A randomised controlled trial.

RR   The relative risk. This is the risk of remission, say, in one group of individuals (eg those receiving treatment) divided by the risk of remission in another group (eg those receiving placebo).

SD   The standard deviation of a set of observations.

$SE(b)$ The standard error of a statistic, b.

$SE(p_1-p_2)$ The standard error of the difference between two estimated proportions

SEM   The standard error of the sample mean; it provides a measure of precision of the estimated mean.

t A particular continuous probability distribution with known and tabulated percentage points so that the P-value relating to the t-test of means can be evaluated from it. Sometimes t is used to denote the test statistic which follows the t-distribution.

T–   An individual whose test result is negative

T+   An individual whose test result is positive

$t_{0.05}$ This is the percentage point or critical value of the t-distribution which gives a total tail area probability of 0·05, i.e. 2·5% of the total area under the curve is contained in the tail to the left of $-t_{0.05}$, and 2.5% is contained in the tail to the right of $t_{0.05}$.

w_i A weight attached to the ith quantity; the weight is used in a calculation to make proper allowance for the relative importance of the quantity.

x This is often used to denote a particular variable, such as the age of an individual. It is commonly used to denote the explanatory or independent variable in a simple regression model.

x_i If x denotes a particular variable, such as age in years, then the subscript, i, indicates the value of that variable for the ith individual in the sample or the population. If there are n individuals in the sample, then the sample values for that variable are ($x_1, x_2, x_3, ...,$ x_n). Alternatively, x_i can denote the ith explanatory variable in a set of explanatory variables in a multiple regression model or in a logistic regression model.

$\bar{x}$ The sample mean of the variable, x (it estimates the population mean, μ). It is pronounced 'x bar', and is equal to the sum of all the values of x in the sample divided by the number of observations, n, in the sample. Hence,

$$\bar{x} = \frac{x_1 + x_2 + x_3 + ... + x_n}{n} = \frac{1}{n} \sum_{i=1}^{n} x_i$$

$\sum_{i=1}^{n} x_i$ This is commonly abbreviated to Σx. The Greek capital letter 'sigma', Σ, indicates that the values of the variable, x, are added up for all the n individuals in the sample, ie from $i = 1$ to $i = n$, so $\sum_{i=1}^{n} x_i = x_1 + x_2 + x_3 + ... + x_n$

y This is commonly used to denote the dependent or outcome variable in a regression model.

Y This is used to denote the predicted or expected value of the outcome variable, y, in a regression model.

Index